KETONES

The Fourth Fuel

Warburg to Krebs to Veech

**The 250-Year Scientific Journey to Find the
Fountain of Youth**

Travis Christofferson

ISBN 13:

CONTENTS

The cover is original artwork by Hope Christofferson
All Illustrations were done by Aubrey Christofferson

We are part of this universe; we are in this universe, but perhaps more important than both of those facts, is that the universe is in us.

—*Neil deGrasse Tyson*

AUTHOR'S NOTE

Before science offered explanations, I'm sure our distant ancestors pondered many questions about their existence and place in the universe and the world around them. What "vital forces" animated the living? What drives motion and thought? Humanities quest to understand how life generates and channels energy is known today as the field of *bioenergetics*. The historical sweep of this collective effort has led to a fascinating new appreciation for a previously maligned metabolic state called *ketosis*. This book is that story.

Our ancestors intuitively understood that life and energy are inextricably woven together—they are one and the same. Everything life does, at the most fundamental level, requires movement, and movement requires energy. Hippocrates claimed the "*vital heat*" to be the function of the *pneuma*, translated to mean *breath*. The pneuma was thought to power the human spirit: our intellect, memories, emotions, fears, and passions. Every lofty manifestation of the human spirit—art, architecture, mathematics, science—was imagined to be powered by the pneuma.

In the abstract the Greeks had captured one of the essential truths of metabolism: everything we do, and for that matter, how we feel—our health and sense of well-being—are all tied to the energy-generating chemical motion that silently and continuously goes on in every one of our 40 trillion cells.

At the epicenter of this story are three remarkable scientists: Otto Warburg, Hans Krebs, and Richard Veech. Although very different as individuals, there was a harmonic resonance to their lives. They all loved gardening, nature and detested having their time wasted. All three, first trained as medical doctors, felt helpless in the role of a physician. Each, then, experienced an awakening—a deep visceral need to understand life on a more fundamental level. They were called to research, and as research scientists, their lives would converge. They all rose to the top of their discipline—a plane of exalted grace that necessitates the best of the human spirit—creativity, artfulness, discipline, logic and inventiveness. Near the end of his autobiography, Krebs mused on what it takes to win a Nobel Prize: "When I ask myself how it came to be that one day I found myself in Stockholm, I had not the slightest doubt that it was because I had had, in Otto Warburg, an outstanding teacher for four years at a critical stage of my development . . . What, then, is it in particular that can be learned from teachers of special distinction? Above all, what they teach is high standards." An outstanding teacher levitates an outstanding student to an even higher plane. The insistence on excellence—the day-in and day-out struggle for perfection—was passed from Warburg to Krebs to Veech.

Their thread of research—handed from one to the other—charted the map of energy metabolism and culminated in a new appreciation of an ancient, auxiliary metabolism that comes installed in our bodies. Their message—their gift to us—is that this metabolic transition, that few are even aware they possess, is so powerfully therapeutic and it has the potential to change the lives of billions—to lift the human spirit in a very real sense.

The arc of this book tracks the historical milestones that led to the discovery of ketone metabolism. The underpinning of ketosis—the *true* reason it is unique—is rooted in biochemistry and physics. As Neil deGrasse Tyson said, "…the universe is in us." The connections between our bodies and the universe are both profound and humbling and have the unique ability to subtly shift our perspective in a way that enhances our appreciation for life. Warburg, Krebs and Veech were dear friends with many physicists over the course of their lives. These relationships influenced their careers and colored their scientific research. I tried to convey some of the many fascinating connections between physics and biology throughout the narrative. We are, in the end, a manifestation of the cosmos *writ large.*

I started writing this book out of a genuine fascination for the subject. However, it quickly morphed into something more urgent. As I write a viral pandemic is sweeping across the globe killing hundreds of thousands in its wake. Surprising to most, the virus, COVID-19, has a much higher death rate among those who suffer from insulin resistance and diabetes—conditions arising from metabolic dysfunction. A solution to these conditions forms the heart of this narrative. As such, the message offered in the pages of this book carries a heightened sense of importance and urgency.

THE VITAL FORCES

B owood House in Wilshire, England was originally a hunting lodge before Lord Shelburne, the Earl of Shelburne, acquired it to be his personal residence. The Georgian country house sat in the middle of a sprawling two-thousand-acre estate in the Wilshire countryside. Behind the walled garden, a pleasure ground of meticulously manicured trees gave way to a gently sloping lawn leading to a sinuous lake. In the summer of 1772, with the demands on his time increasing, Lord Shelburne decided to engage a librarian, a tutor for his children and a general assistant for his own work. He wrote a man of growing reputation named Joseph Priestly offering him the position.

Priestly, the son of a wool cloth maker, had a rough start in life. When Priestly was only a year old he was turned over to his grandfather to raise because his mother was overwhelmed by "having children so fast." He returned home when he was five, after his mother died giving birth to her sixth child. But a few years later, after his father remarried, he was once again sent away, this time to live with his aunt and uncle three miles away in Heckmondwick. The couple had no children. His uncle, "a man of considerable property," died when Joseph was twelve, leaving his aunt a wealthy woman. She recognized Joseph's potential, insisting that her bright nephew attend the finest schools to prepare him for the ministry, which she felt was the most exalted of professions. Young Priestly excelled in school. He quickly mastered Greek, Latin and Hebrew, then at age sixteen, he taught himself French, Italian, German and Arabic. He studied natural philosophy, logic and theology but early on showed a talent for mathematics, chemistry and physics, too. After graduation he took on a series of positions as a minister and teacher at parishes across England. His work afforded him ample time to read, write and conduct chemistry experiments. He published revolutionary works on subjects ranging from metaphysics, politics, theology, chemistry, history and natural philosophy, earning him a reputation as one of England's finest thinkers.

Priestly was both enchanted and conflicted by Lord Shelburne's offer; the salary was much higher than any he received as either a minister or teacher, and the workload would be intentionally light, giving him ample time to conduct experiments in the laboratory Lord Shelburne promised to build for him. Still, he hesitated. He wrote to his dear friend Benjamin Franklin asking for advice. Franklin wrote back: "In the affair of so much Importance to you, wherein you ask my advice, I cannot for want of sufficient premises, advise you what to determine, but if you please I will tell you *how*." Franklin then instructed him to divide a sheet of paper into two columns "writing over the one pro, and over the other con." Franklin instructed him to fill out the columns over the course of a few days and "come to a determination accordingly." Priestly took Franklin's advice. After a few days had passed he noted that the pro column held more "respective weight" than the con column. Priestly wrote Lord Shelburne accepting the position.

Priestly found life at the Bowood house enchanting and soon settled into a comfortable routine. He woke early to write, mid-morning he tutored the children, in the afternoon he advised Lord Shelburne on political affairs, and in the evenings, he conducted his scientific experiments. The first year at the Bowood house passed quickly, and Priestly now found himself spending more and more time in the laboratory. He was particularly captivated by the revolutionary ideas sweeping through the field of chemistry. For over a thousand years it had been accepted that the material world consisted of four elements: earth, wind, water and fire. Newton shattered the four-element paradigm when he demonstrated that what was perceived as white light was actually an amalgam of seven different wavelengths, or colors. The chemists extended Newton's logic proving that "earth," too, could be broken apart into smaller, more elementary components. And now Priestly, with his new and brilliantly designed apparatus, was proving that air (wind) could be deconstructed in a similar manner. Already, he had identified ten new gases. "Air is not an elementary substance, but a composition," declared Priestly.

On August 1, 1774, Priestly woke early. He was anxious to perform an experiment that he had been planning for weeks. Hastily, he dressed and prepared his morning tea. He took a walk through the gardens, sipping tea and collecting his thoughts. The sharp morning songs of the birds stood in contrast to the pillowing scents of summer foliage and the soft morning sun that warmed his face. A few days prior, Priestly had made a curious discovery: He had lit a flame in a large jar, then sealed the container until the flame burned itself out. He then placed a mouse in the container and watched as it soon collapsed, apparently due to the lack of air. Had the flame consumed the life-giving gas within the jar? Inspired, Priestly then repeated that same experiment—depleting the air inside the container with the candle—but this time, in addition to placing the mouse inside the container, he added a mint plant from the garden, sealed the container quickly before gas could be exchanged with the outside air, and set the container in the sunlight. The mouse regained consciousness. Somehow, the combination of plant and sunlight *revitalized* the air and infused the mouse with life force. Additionally, he found that the flame would again burn inside the container after the plant had "restored" the air. Life, flame, and air, Priestly realized, were somehow woven together.

For today's experiment he would again use the sun. He magnified the sunlight spilling through the laboratory's only window onto a small amount of a reddish substance known as mercuric oxide. He then used his apparatus to capture the gas that was released as the mercuric oxide began to burn. For the remainder of the day Priestly would perform a series of experiments with the newly isolated gas. He began with the flame. He noticed that it burned with much more intensity when placed inside a container with the new gas. He again filled the container with the new gas and sealed the mouse inside. Amazingly, when comparing results to those seen with a container filled with normal air, the mouse stayed conscious *four times longer*. This new gas, declared Priestly, was "five or six times as good as common air."

The day had transitioned into night. Candles cast dancing light across the laboratory's walls and cabinets. Outside, the sound of the birds was replaced by crickets chirping under the night sky. Now, intensely focused on learning more about this new gas, Priestly isolated more of it and breathed it deeply into his own lungs. He slowly walked the perimeter of the laboratory, taking careful measure of the effects it had on his body. "The feeling of it in my lungs was not sensibly different from that of common air, but I fancied that my breast felt peculiarly light and easy for some time afterwards. Who can tell but that in time, this pure air may become a fashionable article in luxury. Hitherto only two mice and myself have had the privilege of breathing it," he wrote, late in the night.

Shortly after Priestley's discovery he and Lord Shelburne embarked on a Europe tour, visiting philosophers, dignitaries and scientists in Belgium, Holland, Germany and France. While in Paris, Priestly visited the laboratory of Antoine Lavoisier, a thirty-two-year-old nobleman and chemist. Lavoisier was particularly fascinated by the phenomenon known as *combustion*, loosely defined then as "the act of burning." Indeed, of the four elements, fire had played a transformative role in the story of mankind. By harnessing the power of fire, mankind, in a single leap, transcended the natural world. With fire, mankind was able to transmute wood into heat, food into a more digestible form, and metals into tools. The pre-Socratic Greek, Heraclitus, claimed the soul was a mixture of "fire and water," and the ultimate aim of the soul was to "rid itself of water and become pure fire." The transformative nature of fire led Heraclitus to believe that it was the most fundamental of the four elements. "All things are an interchange for fire, and fire for all things, just like goods for gold and gold for goods." Fire was the only element that could break down and transmute the other elements, its mysterious dual nature as a destructive, transfiguring force and a light-giving, purifying, cleansing force only heightened its mystery. By the eighteenth century, chemists like Priestly felt they finally understood fire. The *phlogiston theory* claimed that within combustible materials there was a common "fire like element," which they called *phlogiston,* that when ignited powered combustion.

When Priestly visited Lavoisier's laboratory in the fall of 1774, Lavoisier was already deeply suspicious that the phlogiston theory was wrong. His own experiments suggested that combustion was not due to some mysterious and invisible element contained within material, but rather due to a *transformation* of the material itself. Part of Lavoisier's genius lay in the negative—he refused to deal in the unknown. If a non-measurable theory was needed to describe a phenomenon—like the mysterious phlogiston was imagined to describe combustion—he doubted it existed at all. "We must trust to nothing but facts: These are presented to us by Nature, and cannot deceive," wrote Lavoisier.

When he meticulously weighed different materials after they were combusted, he noticed a consistent theme: they *gained* mass. To Lavoisier this observation implied that combustion was a process of transformation: the merger of material with air to create a new material. "Nothing is lost, nothing is created, everything is transformed," claimed Lavoisier.

In Lavoisier's laboratory, Priestly excitedly showed the French scientist how to heat mercuric oxide and isolate the new gas. Lavoisier was intensely interested in Priestly's new gas for a specific reason: he suspected that the process of combustion combined material with air, but he didn't know what *specific* gas in the air was combining with the material being combusted. Perhaps, Priestly's lively new gas was the elusive substance within air responsible for combustion. After Priestly departed, Lavoisier isolated himself in his laboratory and conducted a flurry of experiments with the new gas. A year later he published a memoir on the subject unequivocally demonstrating that the new gas—that he now called oxygen—was indeed the "active" component in the air that reacted during combustion. The publication, in a single sweep, spectacularly demolished phlogiston theory and sparked the "chemical revolution" that ushered in modern chemistry.

Yet questions remained unanswered regarding the curious relationship that Priestly had observed between oxygen and the mouse. Priestly observed that oxygen increased the ability to generate energy both in the mouse and himself, but he failed to arrive at an explanation. Indeed, how a living organism generates energy had fascinated, frustrated and confused scholars for centuries. In ancient Egypt it was thought that only some sort of supernatural energy source could power the living. Other than suggesting that food, breath and circulating blood were involved, the Greek philosophers—Plato, Aristotle, and Hippocrates—did little to clarify the issue. The Roman physician Galen claimed that "innate heat" and "spiritedness" were the "vital forces" created by the "pneuma" that was extracted from inhaled air in the lungs. (Respiration comes from the Latin root word "spir" which means breath). The complexity and mystery surrounding the "vital forces" infused from food and breath into living organisms seemed to transcend the knowable world. For over a thousand years the question had hardly advanced beyond the cryptic ruminations of a handful of Greek scholars and mystics. Out of the festering confusion spun a theory called *vitalism* that rapidly swept through early modern Europe. The theory of vitalism was so seductive—so artfully vivid—that it even claimed the great chemist turned biologist, Louis Pasteur. The vitalists claimed that living organisms were imbued with a mystical force that existed on a higher plane that transcended the realm of physical law. (Pasteur was convinced of vitalism because, to date, fermentation—wine making—could only be accomplished by living yeast, and not extracts of dead yeast, invoking a "vital" principle.) It was a theory that was in harmony with, and perhaps bolstered by religious doctrine. "Nothing is so firmly believed as that which we least know," wrote the French philosopher Michel de Montaigue. Still, Lavoisier refused to speculate in the abstract. To Lavoisier, vitalism was the same as the phlogiston theory of combustion—a theory born from ignorance, a theory that conveniently could not be measured, a theory one must take on *faith*.

Lavoisier suspected that the "vital spark" generated by respiration was the same as the combustion of inanimate material—that combustion and respiration were one and the same. Again, Lavoisier turned to what could be measured. His experiments established a powerful corollary: animals inhale oxygen, the "active" component of air responsible for combustion and exhale the same gas that is released from combustion—an inert gas called "fixed air" (later identified as carbon dioxide).

To test his theory—and compare the process of combustion to that of respiration—Lavoisier designed a brilliant series of experiments. For the first experiment he would measure the amount of carbon dioxide released and the heat generated over a fixed amount of time during respiration. To do this he placed a guinea pig inside an enclosed bucket-like apparatus. He then placed the apparatus inside a larger bucket filled with ice. He carefully measured the quantity of carbon dioxide exhaled inside the enclosed chamber while simultaneously measuring the heat released from the guinea pig by measuring the weight of the water collected from the ice that melted. Next, he conducted the same experiment for the combustion of an equivalent amount of carbon. To compare the two, he first determined the amount of carbon, which, upon combustion, would generate the exact same quantity of carbon dioxide as released by the guinea pig in the first experiment. He then compared the heat released by the guinea pig and the combusting carbon by comparing the weight of the water from the melted ice in each experiment. The result confirmed Lavoisier's suspicion: the heat released by the two experiments was the same. "*Ia respiration est donc une combustion*," stated Lavoisier, translated to "respiratory gas exchange is a combustion, like that of a candle burning." The energy of life was not a mystical, unknowable phenomena as the vitalists claimed, proved Lavoisier. Rather, it was simply a "slow combustion."

With Lavoisier's experiment the field of energy metabolism—long muddled by the ambiguous concept of vitalism—leapt forward as it suddenly found clarity. Critically, his experiments illuminated the beginning and the end of the metabolic map: **food + oxygen = energy + carbon dioxide.** Yet, this newfound clarity, like any new discovery, raised entirely new questions. With the beginning and the end established, what lies in the middle? How was the energy from respiration captured in the body? And perhaps even more fundamental: *Where* in the body was respiration taking place?

Lavoisier unrolled the parchment of the metabolic map, drew the first scribbles, and pinned it to the wall. It would be left to others to finish it, however. Lavoisier was an unfortunate victim of the political upheaval during the French Revolution and was beheaded at the age of fifty. Italian mathematician and astronomer, Joseph-Louis Lagrange, said of his death: "It took them only an instant to cut off his head, but France may not produce another such head in a century."

Otto Warburg, born in 1883—eighty-nine years after Lavoisier's death—was one of the explorers who would help chart the map. If this was a calling, Warburg was born and bred for it. Warburg's father was a professor of physics at the University of Berlin and president of the German Physical Society, the oldest and most prestigious physics society in the world. Warburg's father was friends with all the great German physicists and chemists of the era. As regular house guests of the Warburg's, young Otto grew up around Albert Einstein (who became Otto's close friend), Max Planck, Walther Nernst and Emil Fisher, who Warburg would study under while working toward his doctorate in chemistry. Like Lavoisier, Warburg clung to empirical evidence only. His training, philosophy, and internal wiring caused Warburg to fervently—viscerally— reject mystical theories like vitalism. To Warburg, the forces of the universe; thermodynamics, electromagnetism, and energy—all the forces that predictably guided inanimate material—were the same forces that life conformed to. Life, as perceived by Warburg, was a riveting extension of physical law. The field of biology, in general, bothered Warburg. Physics was an edifice built from clean steel; biology, on the other hand, was an unkempt garden—wild and unorderly. Yet, Warburg "came to believe he could bring that same elegant simplicity and clarity [of physics] to the workings of life," wrote a journalist.

Warburg, like Lavoisier, was fascinated by energy. Critically, how does a living organism generate it? And once generated, how is the energy pulsed through the body—powering the senses, thinking and movement? For that matter, how is energy redirected to the hundreds— or thousands—of different cellular processes that must silently work to keep an organism alive?

The chemists and physicists who frequented the Warburg home ingrained in him a triumvirate of thermodynamic laws that elegantly described the biochemical reactions that comprise metabolism. The laws mathematically defined the flow of energy through molecules, atoms, and subatomic particles as they collide, add, subtract and swap parts. The first law of thermodynamics established that energy is never created or destroyed, only *transformed*. In a single moment, the Big Bang infused the universe with all the energy that would ever be. After the Big Bang, this freely drifting cosmic pool of energy went from a calm-sea of evenly distributed energy to a progressively more lumpy distribution—becoming concentrated in things like nebula, stars, black holes, and the bodies of living organisms—if only for a cosmic blink. Lavoisier's experiments showed respiration conformed to the first law: the combustion of mass, as food, released energy that was transformed into a usable form in the body. But what was it transformed into? And *how* was it transformed? These were the questions that captivated Warburg's thoughts. He desperately wanted to know how the first law of thermodynamics applied to the living: *How* was this pool of cosmic energy *captured*, *transformed* and *used* within living organisms?

Through Lavoisier's work, Warburg knew that life generated energy through something called a redox reaction. Chemists had shown that *all* combustion reactions are redox reactions. Redox is short for reduction and oxidation—a dual process describing the shifting distribution of electrons away from one molecule and onto another. A molecule or atom is said to be *reduced* when electrons are transferred to it. It is called a reduction because electrons have a negative charge and therefore "reduce" the amount of charge the molecule previously had. Oxidation is the exact opposite—molecules are *oxidized* when electrons are taken away from them, increasing or creating a positive charge. When a campfire is ignited, electrons are transferred from the hydrogen and carbon in the wood to the oxygen in the air. The take home message is this: Redox reactions can *only* occur as a pair, with one substance oxidized and one reduced. In the campfire example the carbon and hydrogen from the wood are oxidized and the oxygen is reduced. And critically, energy is released from the reaction in the form of heat.

Why is heat released during the process? For that matter, what is heat? Lavoisier mistakenly believed that heat was the vital form of energy that animated the living. Lavoisier imagined heat to be a "subtle liquid"—generated by respiration—that flowed throughout a living organism, infusing it with energy. In the abstract, however, he had captured one of the essential truths of metabolism: energy, like heat, is a form of *motion*. In fact, all forms of energy—mechanical energy, gravitational energy, light energy, electrical, chemical, nuclear and heat energy—though seemingly complex and disparate—when distilled to their essence are nothing more than *motion*. Electrical energy is the *motion* of electrons through a wire, chemical energy is the *motion* of molecules, gravitational energy is the *motion* of an object within a gravitational field. Heat, too, is the energy of motion. But heat is not measured by the motion of an external "substance," as Lavoisier had imagined. Rather, it is motion *internal* to material.

As molecules are broken apart and recombined to form new molecules during combustion it is not a smooth process. It is a ferocious process. Molecular bonds are like taut bungee cords that release their energy when unhooked. In a fire, oxygen combines with the carbon and hydrogen in the cellulose of the wood to form carbon dioxide and water (the water is instantly vaporized in the flame). Picture the water that is created as wood burns. As the hydrogen atoms are stripped from the wood and combine with oxygen atoms from the air they snap together with violent force, causing the newly formed water molecule to spin and vibrate. Imagine taking a metal baseball bat and swinging it at the ground as hard as you can. When the bat hits the ground the energy from the swing is instantly transferred into vibration within the bat, hurting your arms and stinging your hands. This is the same phenomena that creates heat during combustion—the energy of rapidly moving atoms is instantaneously redirected into vibration as new bonds form between atoms. A water molecule is an oxygen atom with two hydrogen atoms on each side. When it vibrates it looks like a person with their arms extended, vigorously waving them up and down. This is heat. The temperature of a material is the measurement of the speed that the molecules within the material are vibrating. The faster the vibration, the hotter the material. In water, if the hydrogen atoms are not vibrating at all, the water forms ice. As we all know from everyday experience, heat tends to transfer itself to nearby objects. The rapidly vibrating carbon dioxide and water from a campfire collide with the surrounding air causing it to vibrate, too. That is the warmth you feel from the campfire—trillions of molecular collisions. Sometimes the transfer is not as gentle. When you touch a hot object, the vibrating atoms act like trillions of molecular buzz saws ripping at the surface of your skin—this is the distinctive feeling and damage of a burn.

Warburg's good friend, Albert Einstein, unveiled another fascinating property of energy. Again, *energy* (a word that gets thrown around pseudo scientifically) is defined as the *movement* of matter. And movement, also called *velocity*, is described by the simple equation: velocity = distance/time, or $V = D/T$.

Rearranging the equation, we can solve for time: $T = D/V$.

This simple equation now holds an essential truth about the universe that is the heart of Einstein's theory of relativity. Looking at the equation reveals a humble but potent understanding: time is only defined by the distance an object travels divided by how fast it's going—in other words, time is *only* defined by movement. Einstein's revelation was that time would be experienced differently depending on the movement of one object relative to another—in other words, time is *relative*. A person traveling very fast in a spaceship will experience the passage of time much more slowly than a person grounded on earth. Einstein's theory of relativity has been proven by atomic clocks with unprecedented accuracy. An experiment using two perfectly synchronized atomic clocks, one placed on a commercial jetliner and the other on the ground, has shown that over time they become unsynchronized, the clock on the jet liner ticks slower than the one on the ground. This is counter to our everyday experience, but nevertheless it is true. Time is a fluid and arbitrary construct—a cognitive trick really—a way for us to sort out a continuum of movement by dividing it into past, present and future.

The equation tells us something else: if movement stops, so does time. Do this thought experiment: Imagine that all the molecules and atoms in your body suddenly stop moving. Every molecule in every cell instantly freezes in place. The atoms that pulse in and out of neurons, firing off the depolarization waves that lead to thoughts, memories, and feelings come to an abrupt halt. Time for you has stopped. What we call consciousness—the continuum of "self"—stops. The aging process stops. And once the material in our body starts moving again, time starts up again. Everything about life—how we age, to how we experience the passage of time—is dependent on energy (movement). This is why animals with faster metabolisms like mice and dogs have much shorter lifespans than animals with slower metabolisms like humans and elephants.

One more fascinating connection between physics and biology. After Einstein proposed that time was relative, he turned to the mysterious force of gravity. Einstein didn't realize it at the time, but the presence of gravity in the universe had extraordinarily far reaching implications. Critically, it would go on to explain the seemingly

impossible existence of life. The second law of thermodynamic reveals an internal messiness to the universe—an
unremitting drive toward disorder. It states that every natural process *increases* the sum total of entropy in the universe. Yet life appears to violate this universal truth. Life is
a curious oasis of order in a universe that craves disorder.
In a universe that relentlessly moves toward disorder, life
appears as a loophole, an exception to a universal rule.
Where does the "order" of life come from?

When the big bang occurred, the universe was at maximum entropy; all the material spilled forth was entirely
unorganized as it expanded outward through the dark
void of space. Yet the universe had other plans. Its material would not remain disorganized for long. There was
an invisible force lurking in the fabric of space and time
that began to mold shape into a shapeless universe. This
gravitational force—that Einstein would later define—
slowly began to work its magic; shaping the material of the
universe into masses with *order*; stars, planets, and moons
began to form that then organized into solar systems and
galaxies. To an omniscient observer, gravity appeared
to be violating the second law of thermodynamics—it
was causing entropy to go "the wrong way." It appeared
an exception to a universal law. "Evidently gravitation
changes the rules of the game in a profound way. A system in which gravitation makes itself felt cannot be considered to be in a state of true thermodynamic equilibrium,
or maximum entropy . . . appearances deceive us," wrote
astrophysicist Paul Davies. Our sun—a highly organized

thermonuclear reactor born from gravity—begin to cast its energy onto a lonely, cold and lifeless planet. The sun bathed the planet with free energy—or *negative entropy*—a wellspring from which *additional order* could spring forth. In other words, the *order* of the sun *flowed* to the earth through free energy. This flow of order was spontaneously transferred to the molecules on earth that captured it and redirected it into life. Life, therefore, is an extension of gravity. "The ultimate source of biological information and order is gravitation," wrote Davies. ". . . the universe is in us," said Neil deGrasse Tyson

The overarching question, then, for the emerging field of biochemistry in the early twentieth century was: *How* is the energy from gravity captured on planet Earth and redirected into life? How does a pool of lifeless atoms unfurl into a living, thinking and breathing creature? With the chemists proving respiration was a redox reaction and the physicists firmly defining energy as the *movement* of material, the challenge for biochemists now was to show how chemical *movement* was coupled to the vital processes of life. Life *is* energy. "Life…is a chemical incident," chemist Paul Ehrlich once quipped. Indeed, an "incident" implies motion. Life is *ordered chemical motion*. Lavoisier revealed respiration to be at the center; the engine spinning the main drive shaft. The firing of neurons, the movement of muscle, the making and recall of memories, the ability to smell, taste, and see—all generated by the movement of electrons, ions, atoms and molecules—must somehow be geared to the main drive shaft. The immediate task—to which Warburg now focused his attention—was revealing how the engine spinning the drive shaft worked. Lavoisier showed the engine was a combustion engine, but Warburg sought a deeper, more inclusive understanding of its internal workings.

Lavoisier had speculated that respiration occurred in the blood but by the end of the nineteenth century researchers established that respiration was occurring within the cells. Still, critical questions remained. Lavoisier established that oxygen was combusting with food, but *how?* The German chemist Felix Hoppe-Seyler established that iron was responsible for delivering oxygen to the cells. Hoppe-Seyler had a powerful visual clue: he could easily observe the shift in the color of blood when oxygen was bound and then released from the iron-containing compound in blood called hemoglobin. The bright red, oxygen-rich blood that had just passed through the lungs gave way to bluish blood as the oxygen was released to the tissues of the body. Biochemists knew that iron was at the heart of this process due to its ability to reversibly bind oxygen. If iron was able to easily attract and release oxygen, then perhaps it was also responsible for attracting oxygen to the site of combustion within the cell. Warburg realized that the cell could capitalize on the oxygen-attracting property of iron, coaxing oxygen to a specific location in the cell, where it was able to combust with the substrates of food. It was as good a place to start as any—so Warburg went looking for iron-containing substances within the cell.

But it was David Keilin, a Polish scientist working at Cambridge, who would make the first stride forward. Keilin, "small in stature but trimly built...," didn't attend school until he was ten years old, due to his struggles with severe asthma. "Although asthma was a constant handicap to him, he was quick and active in his movements and of a cheerful disposition," wrote a colleague. Keilin and Warburg were opposite in every way except their unquestionable brilliance. Warburg was arrogant, stern and demanded respect (he once fired a student on the spot because he felt he didn't greet him with enough respect.) Keilin, on the other hand, was quirky, gentle, self-effacing and humble. Keilin never sought awards, Warburg expected them.

Keilin used a technique known as spectroscopy. In short, spectroscopy uses electromagnetic radiation (x-rays, radio waves, infrared rays and visible light) to probe the structure of atoms and molecules. At the atomic level, atoms interact with light in a unique and measurable way. Individual atoms—and the bonds in between atoms—absorb energy in discrete packets, or "quanta" (this quality is the basis behind quantum mechanics). As such, each atom and each molecule has a unique spectrographic signature—a "barcode" based on the specific wavelengths of light absorbed, referred to as *banding*. Spectroscopy held the surreal ability to peer deep into the bowels of the universe—astronomers had begun making use of this unique quality of matter analyzing the spectrographic signature from interstellar objects like stars and nebulae to determine exactly what gases the objects were made of.

On a smaller scale, emerging spectrographic technology allowed biochemists like Keilin to probe the contents within cells, uncovering the molecules that were hidden inside the cell and discovering new molecules. Keilin had isolated a curious substance from the tissues of flies that produced a unique four-banded spectrum. The four bands were slightly different from the spectrum generated from the fly's blood, hinting that they represented a molecule similar to iron-containing hemoglobin, but subtly different. He then looked at the contents of yeast cells which also respire yet have no blood. The same curious four-banded spectrum emerged. To learn more, he put yeast extract into a test tube with water and vigorously shook the mixture. When he stopped shaking and looked for the bands they were gone. But, interestingly, the bands reappeared a few seconds later. For Keilin, the puzzling disappearance and reappearance revealed a clue. For the banding to disappear the *structure* of the molecule *had* to have changed. Perhaps, he reasoned, the vigorous shaking dissolved oxygen from the air into the water, spurring respiration to start. With respiration now humming along, oxygen would be bound to the molecule, Keilin reasoned, changing its structure and thus its banding pattern. This would account for the disappearance of the bands after he shook the mixture. However, once the dissolved oxygen was used up and respiration came to a halt, there would be no oxygen bound to the molecule, again revealing the four bands he had originally observed. The corollary to Keilin's observation was the shift in color of blood as hemoglobin bound and then released oxygen. "I must admit that this first visual perception of the intracellular respiration process was one of the most impressive spectacles I have witnessed in the course of my work," wrote Keilin.

He then tested to see how widespread the substance or substances were. If he had truly found the site of cellular respiration, he would expect to see it conserved across the animal kingdom. Indeed, everywhere he looked the four bands appeared: from bacteria and yeast, to plants, sponges and everything finned, winged and hooved. By now, Keilin strongly suspected that the bands represented the long-sought-after site of cellular respiration, but he needed more proof. If indeed the substance was involved in respiration one could expect it to be more concentrated in tissues that required more energy, reasoned Keilin. To test his theory, he compared the energy-intensive flight muscle of birds and insects to tissues that required less energy. The results confirmed what he suspected: the banding of the flight muscles were much more intense than the bands from the less energy-intensive tissues.

Keilin then devised a crafty experiment to determine if the four bands represented one or multiple molecules. (He could not yet tell if the bands came from one compound or four compounds, again, because every molecule has a unique spectrographic signature.) To do this, he smeared yeast extract across a slide and watched the absorption bands as the extract dried out. The idea was this: if there was more than one type of molecule, then due to differing structures, they would likely dry at different rates—just like clothes made of different materials dry at different rates when hung on a line. If all the bands disappeared at once, he could be confident the four bands were the signature of a single type of molecule. If, however, they disappeared at different times then he could be confident there were multiple compounds. As he waited, a pattern soon emerged: band A disappeared first, then band B, and finally bands C and D faded simultaneously— the pattern suggested the existence of three separate compounds. Keilin decided to call them cytochrome a, b and c (cytochrome for "colored pigment").

Keilin was confident that he had discovered the elusive site of cellular respiration. Yet to make the claim definitively, he had to prove that one or all of the cytochromes underwent the actual act of combustion and reacted with oxygen. Despite his efforts, he could not conceive of an experiment to accomplish this. It was simply too technically challenging for his time. This is where the story of bioenergetics again paused. This pause troubled Warburg. Keilin was an entomologist and parasitologist who had stumbled sideways into biochemistry. Warburg, however, was a thoroughbred biochemical experimentalist. If anyone could creatively design the experiment to move the science forward it was him. But he needed help.

Luck would prove to be on his side. In the winter of 1926, Warburg met a Jewish physician turned scientist named Bruno Mendel during a dinner party at the home of Albert Einstein. Warburg explained to Mendel the current state of his field—in particular, the standstill in locating the site of cellular respiration. As the evening came to an end Mendel and Warburg promised to stay in contact to exchange ideas and experiments. A few weeks later, during one such phone call, Warburg lamented that he didn't have enough assistants to carry out all of his experimental ideas. Mendel said he could help. He knew a brilliant and hardworking physician who desperately wanted to do research but had yet to find funding. Warburg, despite his reservations on hiring a relatively inexperienced assistant, took Bruno's recommendation and telephoned Dr. Hans Krebs to set up an interview.

LOCATING THE "VITAL SPARK"

Hans Adolf Krebs was born on August 25, 1900 in Hildesheim, Germany. Hans's father, Georg Krebs, was a successful Jewish physician, yet the Krebs family lived a modest lifestyle. Hans's father held majority influence over the household, emphasizing discipline, culture, learning and physical activity. The family tended a beautiful garden of raspberry, strawberry and gooseberry bushes with pear, lime and apple trees lining the perimeter. Music, literature, and chess took up the majority of the time indoors for Hans and his little brother Wolfgang. Outdoors, they swam, rode bikes, climbed trees and took the traditional German Sunday hike with extended family on a meandering gravel path through the wooded hills skirting the village.

Little of Hans's early years hinted of the revolutionary scientist who would later emerge. "I was a good pupil but not outstanding in any subject; it never occurred to me, or anyone else, that I had any special potential," wrote

Krebs. As Hans entered the middle years of grade school, it became obvious that he was a loner. His younger, more gregarious brother played with cousins and friends while Hans would ride his bike alone through the city streets, curl up with a book, or walk through the woods collecting wild flowers to dry and press into an herbarium. Of those years, he would later write that he thought of himself as "a rather unpopular and unattractive boy." Hans's confidence issues were not helped by his father, who often sharply criticized all of his children for being untidy, laughing too much at trivial things, lacking wit and being too shy. He often quoted to his children, with an air of resignation, "You cannot make a silk purse out of a sow's ear." For Hans, who greatly admired his father, these harsh rebukes felt like outright contempt. Rather than rebel or fight back, Hans quietly accepted and internalized his father's criticisms. "My father's critical comments helped me to be modest in assessing my abilities and potential," he would later write.

By the time he was of university age, Hans had decided to follow his father into medicine. Because German medical school training was standardized, it was a common practice for students to switch universities more than once over the course of their education. Taken by the "desire to get away from home and see something else," Hans moved to the University of Freiburg. His "new freedom" in Freiburg was an awakening. Here Krebs thrived. For the first time, he made friends easily and began dating. He enjoyed hiking in the summer and skiing in the winter. It was in Freiburg that a charismatic professor ignited Krebs with a passion for physiological chemistry. The professor stressed the importance of energy metabolism in physiology: "There are no vital functions that take place without chemical motion," said the professor. The concept of all "vital functions" cast from a fountainhead of "chemical motion" deeply resonated with Krebs. Life was chemistry. To understand life, and pathology for that matter, how life went wrong, one must first understand the chemical reactions that animated life at the most basic level.

In the winter of 1923, Krebs graduated from medical school with the overall mark of "very good," the highest mark available in the formal German system. For a newly graduated physician of his time, entering the clinic carried a sense of helplessness. They had few tools to work with. Without antibiotics or chemotherapy, for example, physicians stood by powerless to help as patients died from infections and cancer. Yet a tantalizing series of discoveries harkened of a hopeful new era. A new drug called insulin was being delivered to clinics throughout the world— labeled as a "miracle" for diabetic patients. The discovery of vitamins as essential nutrients promised better health through prevention. As helpless as physicians were, there was now reason for optimism. But it was clear to Krebs the only way to fill the yawning void in meaningful therapies was basic research. "Hans had good reason to feel that he would be able to participate in further advances along these hopeful lines," wrote a colleague.

An associate informed Krebs of a yearlong intensive course in laboratory chemistry designed specifically for MD's who desired to enter research. Krebs's only hesitation was that he would have to ask his father for support for another year. His father reluctantly agreed. Krebs completed the course with "a driving energy," yet "hadn't given much thought to what he might do afterward." A week after completing the course, and with his good friend Mendel's recommendation, Otto Warburg's assistant called to arrange an interview. Krebs was intimately familiar with Warburg's work and reputation—he knew he was a giant in the field of biochemistry.

In December of 1926, Krebs sat nervously in Warburg's office on the top floor of the Kaiser-Wilhelm Gesellschaft, as Warburg entered the room. For thirteen years Warburg had been a "member" of the Gesellschaft, a designation only granted to a handful of exceptional scientists (Einstein was also a member). Members were given a generous salary and absolute freedom in their choice of research, and "no teaching or administrative responsibilities whatsoever." Upon appointment Warburg was told "You will be completely independent. No one will ever trouble you. No one will ever interfere. You may walk in the woods for a few years or, if you like, may ponder over something beautiful." Warburg had been the youngest scientist ever appointed to the institute and remained there his entire career. "I have no doubt that my scientific successes are very largely due to the exceptional measure of freedom and independence which I enjoyed...," wrote Warburg.

Krebs was not a shy, insecure boy anymore. Still, Warburg was an intimidating figure. His steely blue eyes darted back and forth as he reviewed the stack of Krebs's published research papers, without muttering a single word. He paused—Krebs adjusted himself nervously in his chair. "What are your future plans," asked Warburg. Krebs replied that his plan was to go into academic medicine—to teach while continuing to do research. The assistantship with Warburg was a one-year appointment with a modest salary. Warburg informed Krebs that once the assistantship was over, he would be unable to help him find a job as an academic physician because he was so disliked by most universities. You better attach yourself "to some old ass of a professor," he told Krebs. Krebs, however, wasn't concerned. He was ecstatic with the opportunity to learn from one of the best biochemists in the world, even if it was only for a year.

Two weeks later, at 8:00 a.m., the day after New Year's Day, 1926, an elated Krebs entered Warburg's laboratory for the first time. "This is the best job I could have dreamed of," he thought to himself. Krebs was captivated by the raw pleasure of research—to explore the murky border between the known and unknown of biochemistry was as exhilarating to him as it must have been to the great explorers as they charted the rivers, mountains and forests of new continents.

Warburg entered immediately behind him. "Good morning Chief," said another assistant. Everyone in the laboratory called Warburg "Chief"—a nickname that reflected his authoritarian style. The group was expected to arrive at 8:00 a.m. and leave at 6:00 p.m., six days a week. Evenings and Sundays were reserved for data analysis, notebook entries, and literature searches. If you worked in Warburg's laboratory, there was little distinction between your life inside the lab and outside the lab—your research was expected to be your life, anything else would land you out on the street. "Science was the dominant emotion," Krebs would later write.

After the morning pleasantries, Warburg placed Krebs opposite his lab bench and immediately began instructing him on how to use a *manometer*—a glass tube apparatus that could measure the gases emitted by redox reactions from tissue samples. Warburg had designed his own state-of-the-art manometer that operated with unprecedented accuracy. It is somewhat inexplicable that Warburg accepted an assistant as inexperienced as Krebs, much less that he decided to personally train him. But Krebs was a quick student, and in just a few weeks he had become proficient with the apparatus. Warburg then assigned him his first research project. The discovery of the three iron-containing cytochromes by Keilin still loomed large. In Warburg's mind, the first step to prove that the iron-containing cytochromes were the site of cellular respiration—as Warburg strongly suspected—was to prove that cells *required* iron to respire. By April of 1926, Krebs had obtained unequivocal results showing that cellular respiration was indeed dependent on iron, confirming Warburg's instincts. After examining his results, Warburg declared, "Now you have discovered something."

Warburg was now certain that Keilin's cytochromes were somehow involved in cellular respiration. They now faced the daunting task of zeroing in on the individual cytochromes. The next assignment for Krebs was more difficult and would require creativity, ingenuity, and dogged persistence. The task was straightforward: find the cytochrome, or cytochromes, where respiration was occurring. In other words, find the exact location where oxygen was combining with the breakdown products of food.

Krebs dove into the project with unrelenting zeal. Like Keilin, he found the task technically challenging in the extreme. Months of experiments with no answer led to frustration. But, unwilling to give up, they thought of a shrewd experiment that just might tease out the answer. They envisioned a clever expansion of the spectrographic technique that Keilin used to discover the presence of the cytochromes. Perhaps, they reasoned, they could use carbon monoxide as a probe to tease out the location of respiration. It was known that carbon monoxide is structurally similar to oxygen and therefore, when present in the blood could replace oxygen on the iron-binding site in hemoglobin (this is the mechanism behind carbon monoxide poisoning). For Krebs and Warburg's purpose, carbon monoxide had another fortuitous property: when bound to iron, certain wavelengths of light could oust it from the iron-binding site within hemoglobin. Warburg and Krebs realized they could use these properties of carbon monoxide to their advantage. The experiment they proposed went like this: they would bubble carbon monoxide into the tissue sample and halt respiration as the carbon dioxide displaced the oxygen bound to the cytochrome. They would then focus the specific wavelength of light on the tissue necessary to displace the carbon monoxide from the iron in the cytochrome to restart respiration. The changes in the spectrum banding as respiration stopped and restarted, Krebs and Warburg realized, would then reveal the cytochrome or cytochromes where respiration was occurring.

They eagerly recorded the spectrum of each cytochrome as they conducted the experiment from beginning to end: the spectrum bands of cytochromes b and c remained unchanged with the addition and then removal of carbon monoxide, but the bands of cytochrome a had shifted. This was unambiguous proof: The long-sought-after site of respiration was cytochrome a. This experiment would earn Warburg a Nobel Prize in 1931. Nobels are awarded not only for the profound importance of what an experiment reveals about nature, but also for the artfulness of the experiment itself—Warburg's 1931 Nobel met both standards. When Warburg learned of his Nobel Prize, his response was: "It's high time."

Warburg and Krebs's Nobel Prize-winning experiment now answered the question of *where* respiration was occurring in the cell, but it left many other questions unsolved.

Chiefly, if cytochrome a was the site of respiration, what was the purpose of the other cytochromes—cytochromes b and c? Moreover, how were all the widely variable components of food—fats, protein, and carbohydrates—all combusted by a single cytochrome? Keilin (who corresponded with Warburg frequently) proposed a possible solution: perhaps, he reasoned, food was broken down into its most elementary form—single hydrogen atoms. Perhaps, the hydrogen atoms had their electrons stripped off and were then passed from one cytochrome to the next, like an electrical current moving through a wire, until they reached cytochrome a, the end of the line. There, the electrons reacted with oxygen, completing the process of respiration. Indeed, the fact that each cytochrome contained an iron atom strengthened Keilin's hypothesis—chemists knew metal atoms like iron conduct the flow of electrons with ease.

Warburg vehemently disagreed with Keilin's proposal. Warburg refused to speculate—maintaining one could only conclude what the data revealed. He felt there was simply no evidence to say that cytochromes b and c were involved in respiration at all. He contended that the components of food were respired in a single step, on cytochrome a. Still Keilin disagreed, based on intuitive reasoning. "It is inconceivable to ascribe the whole of the respiratory system to the activity of only one type of enzyme to the exclusion of the other type," said an exasperated Keilin. Warburg shot back in his Nobel Lecture: "It is still not possible to answer the question [regarding the role of the other cytochromes]." Perhaps due to his arrogance; perhaps just to frustrate Keilin, Warburg often referred to cytochromes b and c as "degenerate ferments." Framing them like an appendix—a vestige of our evolutionary past—evolutionary baggage that at one time served a purpose but was no longer relevant.

What was originally intended to be a one-year appointment in Warburg's laboratory had extended to nearly four years. Krebs didn't appear to be in a hurry to find a new job, but for reasons not obvious to Krebs, Warburg was growing increasingly impatient with him. He made it clear it was time for Krebs to move on. In the summer of 1928, Krebs made arrangements to attend the Nineteenth International Congress of Physiology in Boston, the most prestigious conference at the time with over 1,000 scientists from 35 countries scheduled to attend. On the first of August, Krebs boarded a brand new, state-of-the-art German ocean liner for what would be a calm five-day journey across the Atlantic. The whirlwind trip was electrifying for Krebs. He attended inspiring lectures. He had stimulating conversations and established numerous contacts with fellow scientists at the conference. He spent time in a colleague's laboratory at Harvard. He traveled to New York, stopping at Princeton to give a guest lecture. In New York he visited the laboratories of colleagues, roamed through museums, and even watched his first "talking" film, *Sonny Boy.*

Krebs returned from his trip intellectually inspired and percolating with creative energy. Upon his return to the lab, rather than infecting Warburg with his new found enthusiasm, Krebs's excitement seemed to have the opposite effect—it was clear that Warburg was displeased that Krebs left the conference without any immediate job prospects. "You must be gone from here by April first," Warburg said. Krebs was taken aback. He had assumed he could stay as long as he proved himself useful. The growing tension seemed to be coming from the unequivocal authoritarian manner in which Warburg ran his laboratory. With Krebs's growing skill and confidence, he had begun suggesting experiments and even questioning Warburg on occasion. For Krebs, the position he now found himself in spoke of a deeper internal tension. "Deeply woven into the texture of Hans Krebs early life was a tension between dependence and autonomy, between conformity to expectations and creative initiative," wrote his biographer.

Moreover, it had become apparent that their research interests had sharply diverged. Both were still intensely captivated with discovering how cells generate energy, but each wanted to explore different pieces of the problem. Warburg's interest in respiration was limited: for him, it would be enough to uncover what food molecules feed into the system at the beginning and how these molecules were then combusted with oxygen at the end. Krebs, however, was increasingly captivated by the yawning void in the middle of the process: What series of linked reactions connected the beginning to the end? Now it was clear: if

Krebs was to become an independent investigator, it was time to move on. "During my last few months in Warburg's laboratory, I did a great deal of heart-searching about the kind of career I should aim at," Krebs would write later.

In the summer of 1931, Krebs landed a well-paying job in Freiburg. As it was for him in medical school, the enchanting medieval village nestled in the Black Forest would again be a revelation, declaring he finally felt "completely free, for the first time, to follow my own ideas on research and choose my own subject." In Freiburg, he resumed practicing medicine. The job required him to maintain clinical duties during the day, which he increasingly enjoyed. He would then retreat to the laboratory in the evening and into the night. Here Krebs flourished; he felt a deep satisfaction from helping patients during the day, and, at night, still felt the stir of discovery that research had always given him. But something had changed. He no longer had to ask his father for money and he no longer needed Warburg as a mentor; he was now a competent medical doctor and a competent research scientist. Both his father and Warburg could be harsh and unforgiving. Yet Krebs would never speak ill of either of them. He later described Warburg as "the most remarkable person I had ever known." For Krebs, Warburg's faults— arrogance, pettiness and combativeness—were eclipsed by his good qualities—brilliance, eccentricity and independence. "Whenever people who knew him were together, their conversation turned sooner or later to the subject of his personality. What fascinated people, apart from his penetrating intelligence . . . was his intellectual honesty and straightforwardness, his singularity of purpose and his industry, the wit and humour of his pertinent comments on affairs—scientific or other, his generosity in helping people in the laboratory, and his eccentricities. Those who knew him well were very ready to overlook weaknesses, his touchiness and his resentfulness, his prejudices and his harshness against those whom he regarded unjustifiably as his 'enemies,'" Krebs later wrote.

But Krebs had moved on. Every question was now his to explore, every experiment his to design, every discovery his to claim. For the first time, Krebs was his own man.

Now a completely independent researcher, Krebs was free to investigate any interests he desired. He turned to a problem that had vexed biochemists for decades: the metabolism of *proteins*. Protein plays a pivotal role in life. In the cell, proteins do the heavy lifting. If DNA is the CEO calling the shots, then proteins are the legions of blue-collar workers keeping the business running. Proteins provide structure, build muscle, and catalyze metabolic reactions. They act as receptors, hormones and couriers of information, relaying messages from outside the cell back to DNA—signaling which genes to turn on and which ones to turn off. DNA provides the code to manufacture cellular proteins—the *message* contained within each gene is translated into *action* by proteins. One gene equals one protein. Proteins are made up of a chain of smaller sub-units called amino acids. The pattern, or "code" of four molecules called *base pairs* in a given gene, determines the order of the amino acids in its corresponding protein. A unit of three base pairs, called a *codon*, calls for one of the twenty amino acids. The codon is the Rosetta Stone of biology—translating the language of DNA into that of proteins. For a gene to manufacture a protein, first, large, industrial-like proteins travel along the gene, reading each codon as they go and translating the information into a messenger molecule called messenger RNA (mRNA). The mRNA serves as an intermediary between DNA and pro-teins, like a pigeon carrying a letter. Another large protein then attaches to mRNA, reading it codon by codon, pick-ing out the amino acids designated by each codon, and stitching them together to form a protein. This is the code of life. The flow of information in biological systems is a one-way street from DNA to RNA to protein. Francis Crick called this flow of information "The central dogma of life."

There is an old saying in biology: "structure equals function." The structure of your hand, with its oppos-ing thumb, grants it the functionality to grab objects. The same concept holds true at the nanoscale environ-ment of proteins. The structure determines whether a protein acts as an enzyme facilitating a chemical reac-tion, a receptor that binds insulin, a hormone, a muscle fiber, or something else. Proteins are first manufactured as a linear chain of amino acids, but in the aqueous envi-ronment of the cell, proteins instantly fold up into their most "comfortable" configuration. The forces that guide the folding into the protein's final shape are common to everyday experience. When you drip olive oil into a pot of water the droplets don't disperse, they stay huddled up in a circular form in the water. But if you put sugar in the water it dissolves instantaneously. The chemical characteristics of individual amino acids are the same as the olive oil and the sugar—the oil-like, hydrophobic (water-hating) amino acids huddle up together on the inside of the protein, trying to stay away from the water. The sugar-like, hydrophilic (water-loving) amino acids prefer to freely associate with the aqueous environment of the cell and remain on the outside of the protein. These two forces, then, guide the collapse of proteins into their final shape.

DNA is an information storage molecule—it is our hard drive. The sweep of evolution—played out over millenniums—shuffles the four base pairs in DNA through the process of random mutation thus altering the codons and causing different amino acids to be incorporated into proteins. Perhaps, for example, a hydrophobic amino acid is introduced in place of a hydrophilic amino acid in a given protein. Now, the protein folds into a different shape, changing its functionality. Perhaps the protein doesn't function as well, resulting in a less "fit" organism; perhaps the change is catastrophic, and the protein is rendered nonfunctional and the organism dies, either way, the mutation is filtered from the gene pool. Maybe the protein functions better, conveying a survival advantage to the organism and the mutation becomes conserved in the gene pool. This is evolution at the molecular level. Evolution acts on DNA in a removed, apathetic and cold manner, randomly swapping letters in a code. Proteins, however, are the front line of evolution, the proving grounds where new machinery gets tested in an unforgiving and binary manner: its either *better* or *worse*. To see the structure of a protein is to witness the unfathomable complexity and beauty of life: Primary structures collapsing into symmetrically repeating secondary patterns; helixes, globular formations and sheets; that then collapse into functional tertiary structures. Researchers have recently uncovered a new class of proteins called *Intrinsically Disordered Proteins.* These astonishing proteins are evolution at its most wonderous—proteins with a structure that is an ordered *disorder*; a planned randomness that allows proteins to achieve multiple functionalities. These proteins eschew the normal rigid structural patterns of proteins, rather, they have an engineered fluidity; a loose arrangement that builds in flexibility, allowing them to snap from a chaotic arrangement into a functional structure as needed. As relentless, apathetic and unforgiving as Darwinian evolution is, its end result is an unfathomable display of artful, nanoscale engineering—tens of thousands of proteins, their structure sculpted over eons of life and death, pain and elation, that magically—in perfect harmony—take a pool of inanimate atoms and organize them into a living, breathing, thinking creature.

The biochemists of Krebs era had discovered that protein could also act as a metabolic fuel if needed. When a person eats a protein-rich meal, hydrochloric acid and digestive enzymes immediately go to work breaking the protein down into its constituent amino acids that are then absorbed and distributed to every cell in the body. The pool of amino acids is then reassembled into new cellular proteins as needed. However, in contrast to carbohydrates and fat, amino acids cannot be stored. Therefore, an excess of amino acids is either processed directly for energy or converted into glucose or fat. This processing of excess amino acids requires the removal of the nitrogen-containing amino group, thus creating *ammonia*. This creates a problem for the cell: ammonia is very toxic and needs to be disposed of immediately.

In the 1930s, however, biochemists didn't know how the body rid itself of ammonia. The problem was too daunting for most researchers to consider. Even the "Chief" thought it was too experimentally difficult to approach. In Freiburg, inspired by his new freedom, Krebs orchestrated a series of brilliant experiments that uncloaked a remarkably efficient waste-disposal cycle that he called the *urea cycle*. Krebs showed that ammonia combines with a compound called ornithine which is then cycled through a series of reactions converting it into a molecule called *urea*. Urea is then cleaved from ornithine and excreted as waste in the urine—thus regenerating ornithine and starting the cycle all over again—a beautifully evolved self-perpetuating waste-disposal process.

With the urea cycle, Krebs had revealed the first example of a complete metabolic cycle. For Krebs, it was a glimpse into the remarkable economy of nature. A metabolic cycle was a beautiful thing to behold—an extraordinary economical solution to solve a metabolic need. A cycle, as opposed to a linear series of reactions, allowed for more regulatory control. It had built-in flexibility—if needed, it could spin faster to remove more waste. The cycle could act like a central hub, with molecules pulled out to enter into other metabolic processes to be used for other purposes—like a roundabout intersection with cars continuously entering and exiting, fanning out to any number of near and distant locations. And cycles could be geared together, swapping molecules back and forth as needed to meet the metabolic requirements at the moment.

On April 30, 1932, the same day the paper on the urea cycle was published, Krebs received a telegram from his dear friend Bruno Mendel: "Congratulations on your very beautiful work. Warm Regards, Bruno Mendel." Even Warburg was impressed, as was Hans' father, whose respect and adoration Krebs still craved. Krebs had now established himself as a top-ranked biochemist. Indeed, everything was going right for Krebs; he loved his work and his surroundings in Freiburg, but unbeknownst to him, dark clouds were gathering.

Although he was mostly insulated from the economic problems stirring in post—World War I Germany, Krebs was aware of the growing social unrest and the rising influence of the Nazi party, led by Adolf Hitler. He had read enough of Mein Kampf to know what this meant for him as a Jew. He heard the rumors that some Jews were already leaving Germany. Krebs, however, remained optimistic, holding on to the hope that "it would sort itself out."

This optimism was extinguished all at once when, on January 30, 1932, it was announced that Adolf Hitler had become the new chancellor of Germany. Now Krebs' future in Germany rested on the hope that those around Hitler could constrain him. Yet it was becoming clear that life had dramatically changed. Even in the peaceful village of Freiburg, men in Nazi uniforms seemed to sprout up from nowhere. Political demonstrations and radio broadcasts of Nazi propaganda became more and more frequent and frightening. Four weeks into the new regime, a lone arsonist set Reichstag (home of the German Parliament) on fire. Hitler seized the opportunity, declaring the fire was a communist plot to take over Germany, and invoked emergency powers. With the escalating unrest and paranoia, Hitler quickly maneuvered himself into absolute dictatorial power. Then on April 7, the Law for the Restoration of Career Civil Service was issued by the Nazi Minister of the Interior. The law stated that those of "non-Aryan" descent were to be immediately removed from civil service jobs.

The next day, news of the new law was on the front page of newspapers around the world. A worried former colleague of Krebs who was now working at Cambridge University in England, wrote to Krebs offering him a position. Still, Krebs remained strangely optimistic despite the fact that many of his Jewish colleagues, including Einstein, had already fled Germany: "I believe that your judgement of the situation from a distance appears darker than it is at the moment," Krebs wrote back. "Here in Freiburg, no one at the University, so far as I know, has been dismissed." Four days later, Krebs received another blow struck by a note in his mailbox: "By order of the academic rectorate I inform you, in accordance with ministerial order A Nr. 7642, that you are on leave until further notice."

Now unable to work—perhaps trying to forget the unrest swirling around him that was beyond his control— he packed his notebooks into a backpack and rode his bike deep into the Black Forest. His intent was to relax, write and think. He rode to the resort town of St. Peter and checked into the Pension Schar, an idyllic hotel with cascading valleys off to one side and steep mountains rising on the other; far in the distance the majestic peaks of the Swiss Alps could be seen. Here, Krebs took leisurely hikes, sunbathed, and began to write review articles on amino acid and fatty acid metabolism. It was a welcome respite from the ominous political affairs now seizing Germany. Krebs was happiest surrounded by nature with his thoughts lost entirely to the chemistry of life. Unfortunately, his respite would not last long. A few day later he received a letter sent directly to the hotel: "By order of the Minister of Culture and Instruction, the State Commissioner, we hereby inform you that in preparation for the execution of the laws for the reconstruction of the professional service, you are relieved of you present employment, and you are given notice that your service will be terminated on July 1, 1933." The letter then instructed Krebs to "certify your receipt of this notice by signing the enclosed form, and that you return this certification immediately."

Krebs packed his belongings and rode his bike back into Freiburg to discover his laboratory was barred from entry. It was finally clear to Krebs that his life was in danger; he could no longer delay in leaving Germany. Warburg, despite some Jewish heritage of his own, did not bear the brunt of antisemitism due in part to his reputation, but it was also known that Hitler was terrified of cancer and Warburg was considered Germany's leading cancer researcher. Warburg wrote to Krebs, offering him a position as a "guest scientist" but admitted it was probably better if he left Germany all together. His colleagues at Cambridge were hurriedly trying to find a position for him but bureaucratic red-tape was slowing the process. Finally, on May 31, Krebs decided he couldn't wait any longer. He convinced the hospital staff to allow him to pack up his laboratory equipment and have it shipped to England. On June 19, he boarded the 11:00 am train for Strasburg and left mainland Europe behind for good.

Once in England, Krebs received good news—he had been awarded a grant by the Rockefeller Foundation. This made it much easier for his advocates at Cambridge to secure him a position. As he settled in, he was immediately enchanted by the English culture. Warburg was a fervent Anglophile and often made trips to England to buy riding kits, antique furniture and suits from Savile Row. "The English tolerate headstrong and eccentric people—like me," said Warburg. Warburg felt the numerous honors and degrees bestowed upon him in Germany were a waste of his time, but he was proud to have received an honorary degree from Oxford. "He loved the keeping up of traditions and the dignified pomp and circumstance of the ceremonial which he experienced when he was given an honorary degree at Oxford in 1965. 'England is the last bastion of the old Europe,' said [Warburg]," recalled a colleague.

Krebs could now see the attraction. He described the thriving intellectual atmosphere at Cambridge as a "hive of activity." He found the bustling culture and warm hospitality of the English as suiting him "down to the ground." A year later, Krebs secured a more permanent position at the University of Sheffield in Yorkshire, with a higher salary and a larger laboratory. Here, Krebs again turned to the still-festering question of energy metabolism: How is food ultimately respired to create energy?

As with the urea cycle, Krebs was more interested in uncloaking the entire process from beginning to end. The untidy nature of energy metabolism still bothered him. To Krebs, the state of the field looked like a collection of scattered puzzle pieces. Researchers had identified many individual reactions: glucose and amino acids could be converted to other metabolites; fats appeared to be chopped up into bite-size molecules consisting of two carbon atoms. The problem was that most of the reactions weren't connected to anything; they were just left dangling in space—an arbitrary collection of biochemical reactions floating in the pages of textbooks and journals. To read a biochemistry textbook in the 1920s and 30s felt less like a scientific discipline and more like the ravings of a mad man—random letters slurred together that formed neither words, sentences or paragraphs. Biochemistry desperately needed researchers to establish order; to explain *how* the collection of known reactions were linked together. The fundamental tenet of biochemistry—the end goal—is to illuminate an atlas of metabolic pathways: a linked series of reactions that form pathways that then branch, merge, and cycle as they carry out the functionality of life. "The final goal of physiological chemistry," wrote one of Krebs's professors, "is to present a scheme that puts together a series of unbroken equations of all the reactions from the foodstuffs which continuously supply to the organism its energy needs, all the way to the slag that again leaves the organism as energyless final oxidation products." For the time being, however, the map Lavoisier unrolled long ago consisted mostly of expansive voids with a few a smatterings of land. Krebs had stitched together the reactions involved in the generation of urea from beginning to end; now he set about to do the same for respiration.

With the dark clouds of Hitler's Germany behind him, Krebs could now focus all his energy on mapping the intermediate metabolism of respiration. The beginning of respiration was mostly illuminated thanks to one of Warburg's former students, Otto Meyerhof, who worked one floor below Warburg at the Kaiser-Wilhelm Gesellschaft in Berlin. (It was fitting to Warburg that Meyerhof worked below him, as Warburg was often heard insulting his abilities). Meyerhof had illuminated the first steps in carbohydrate (glucose) metabolism. Experimenting with muscle tissue that was sliced thin enough to allow oxygen to freely diffuse into the cells, Meyerhof stimulated the muscle to contract and mapped out the series of reactions as glucose was pulled from storage and burned as fuel. Meyerhof noted that when muscle burned glucose without oxygen present, lactic acid formed. Conversely, when muscle burned glucose in the presence of oxygen, two molecules of *pyruvate* formed. Meyerhof's pathway led to two different end products: the anaerobic pathway (without oxygen) led to lactic acid and the aerobic (with oxygen) pathway ended with pyruvate. Meyerhof established the beginning and end of the glucose-burning pathway but another German biochemist, Gustav Embden, filled in the middle. Working in a laboratory in Frankfort, Embden showed that the pathway, which would come to be known as *glycolysis*, consisted of ten reactions in total.

The pathway Meyerhof and Embden unveiled was unique for several reasons—first, it was conserved across the animal kingdom, essentially the same in *all* living organisms, from bacteria to humans. This implied the pathway was both ancient and fundamental to life.

Second, the pathway could produce energy with or without oxygen. This suggested the pathway may have evolved before the earth's atmosphere was oxygenated—some 2.5 billion years ago—when the *only* biochemical solution to energy production for the single-celled organisms that dominated the planet was one without oxygen. Also curious was the fact the pathway only used carbohydrate. Somewhere, in life's ancient past, glucose was selected as the vital fuel. Although life would eventually evolve the ability to use other fuel sources, this fundamental (and ancient) reliance on glucose as a fuel was established as an evolutionary starting point—a biochemical pillar for the relentless engine of evolution to begin building upon—a vestige of our evolutionary past. The *glycolytic pathway* is where Meyerhof's and Embden's contribution ended—where the metabolic map again went dark—the fate of the end products of glycolysis, lactate and pyruvate, remained unknown.

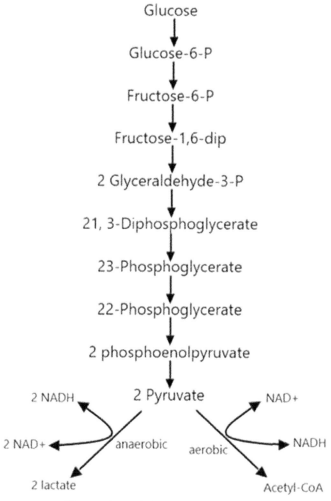

Illustration of the Glycolytic Pathway

As Krebs looked at the state of the map of metabolic reactions making up respiration, he considered the other points of illumination. A Hungarian-American biochemist, Albert Szent-Gyorgyi, had discovered that certain compounds were formed but then disappeared at the same rate that carbohydrate was consumed. This hinted that they were "intermediates" (a.k.a. metabolites) in the respiratory process—chemical reactions in-between the general equation Lavoisier had established: food + oxygen = carbon dioxide + energy. Two German biochemists then discovered more intermediates: a molecule called citric acid was converted in two steps to a molecule called alpha-ketoglutarate.

Krebs was convinced that all of these intermediates were somehow linked, but he wasn't sure how. Krebs closed his eyes and considered what he already knew. Single molecules of glucose were separated, one at a time, from glycogen (a chain of glucose molecules used for storage). Next, glucose was shunted down the glycolytic pathway, step by step, arriving at pyruvate. Then Krebs had his eureka moment. Those that came before him had only envisioned metabolic pathways as linear, like the glycolytic pathway. Krebs's genius lay in imagining it as a *cycle*—like the urea cycle that he had elucidated in Freiburg. In his mind he bent the series of reactions from a straight line into a circle: citrate -> isocitrate -> alpha-ketoglutarate -> succinate -> fumarate -> malate -> oxaloacetate. The loop just needed to be closed, imagined Krebs. And he then imagined a way to close it: pyruvate. All at once this snapped together Meyerhof's glycolytic pathway with a cyclical series of intermediate reactions. Now he had to prove it. The experiment itself was incredibly simple. He paired *oxaloacetate*, the molecule at the end of the chain, with *pyruvate*, the molecule at the end of the glycolytic pathway, to see if they reacted to form *citrate*, the molecule at the beginning of the cycle. "So I used suspensions of minced pigeon flight muscle to test whether oxaloacetate and pyruvate together formed citrate, and found that they did." He had done it—he had closed the loop. The reaction: pyruvate + oxaloacetate = citrate, connected the glycolytic pathway with a cycle of intermediate reactions. Science crawls its way forward by *connection*; Darwin *connecting* biological traits to the dynamically changing environment, Copernicus *connecting* the revolving planets to the sun, Newton *connecting* a falling apple to gravity—Krebs had connected a seemingly unconnected series of metabolic reactions into a unified whole.

By 1953, the year that Krebs was awarded a Nobel Prize for his "Krebs cycle," the field of biology had woken from a long slumber; suddenly it was crackling, electric—alive. One hundred miles to the southeast, in Cambridge, Watson and Crick had just unveiled the structure of DNA to the world—the molecule at the center of the biological universe. Simultaneously, across the Atlantic, American developmental biologists Robert Briggs and Thomas King cloned the first vertebrate by transplanting nuclei (DNA) from a fully mature, differentiated cell into egg cells with the nucleus removed—crushing the century old assumption that once a cell type was established, the DNA was "fixed"—demonstrating a remarkably counterintuitive flexibility of the genome. A year later, the three-dimensional structure and synthetic pathway of cholesterol was revealed. The year after that, the enzyme responsible for replicating DNA was discovered. Yet, if one looked closely, the Krebs cycle was the literal wellspring behind the biological revolution. It accounted for the substrates and the energy needed for *all* the remarkable discoveries taking place in biology: the energy spun from the Krebs cycle was needed to replicate DNA as cells divided, to build a multicellular organism from a single nucleus, to drive the synthetic pathways that manufacture vitamins and cholesterol—indeed, *all* cellular processes were dependent on the *chemical motion* of energy metabolism—with the Krebs cycle rotating at the center.

The cycle Krebs elucidated would go on to become the most famous metabolic pathway in biochemistry. It would become known by many names: The citric acid cycle, the tricarboxylic acid cycle, and the Krebs cycle. The Krebs cycle is the cell's vital hub of metabolic activity. Its fame is born from the cycle's central importance in metabolism. Its importance is owed to the fact it is simultaneously two things at once: a catabolic cycle (breaking down molecules for energy) and an anabolic cycle (synthesizing new molecules). As the cycle spins, energy is extracted from the initial substrates to be used elsewhere in the cell. Additionally, the cycle serves as a source of metabolites, whirling them from the cycle to serve as substrate for other critical biosynthetic pathways. For the cell, the Krebs cycle is both the fire and the emerging phoenix. One author summed up its essential nature: "You might say I've become an unwilling expert on the Krebs cycle. It's vital to my existence. Life and death, really. That tends to focus one's attention . . . It's the cellular engine. A gift of evolution. How our bodies convert carbohydrates, proteins and fats into carbon dioxide, water and energy. When it stops working, we die."

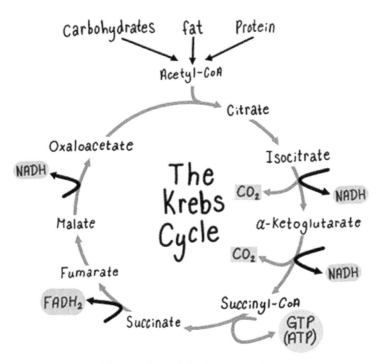

Illustration of the Krebs Cycle

Biochemists like Meyerhof and Krebs were able to link together the series of reactions exposing the pathways comprising human metabolism, but that didn't explain *how* the reactions were occurring. The metabolic map was punctuated with chemical reactions—molecules changing from one form into another—but what *caused* the reactions to take place? It was highly unlikely that they were happening spontaneously. Scientists suspected something must be enabling, or *catalyzing* the reactions.

The concept of a catalyst was first proposed by a Scottish scientist named Elizabeth Fulhame in 1794. A catalyst, claimed Fulhame, was a substance that increases the rate of a chemical reaction without itself undergoing any permanent chemical change. A catalyst could be thought of like a ferry, shuttling people across an otherwise uncrossable river over and over again. Early on, chemists noticed that certain metals could speed up combustion reactions and remain unchanged after the reaction sputtered to a halt. The idea of catalyst in biology was suggested by the great Louis Pasteur to explain the "vital force" as yeast magically transformed the sugar in grapes into wine. A German scientist then coined the word "enzyme," derived from the Greek word for "In Yeast," to describe Pasteur's "vital force." But it would take until 1926—the year Krebs entered Warburg's laboratory—for an American chemist named James Sumner to isolate an enzyme from living tissue. Sumner's discovery was an epiphany in the field of biochemistry. The reactions that animated life—Meyerhof's and Krebs's pathways—were not spontaneously set ablaze like Lavoisier's candle. The reactions were carefully facilitated by protein enzymes manufactured within the cell. The "vital spark" of life burns by subtly catalyzing thousands of chemical reactions that would not normally occur. Enzymes manipulate chemistry—they allow life to exist on a controlled chemical plane just above a pool of inanimate molecules that have no interest in reacting with one other. And unlike the catalysts that chemists were familiar with—ones that simply set a reaction into motion—like tapping the first domino in a row—life's manipulation of chemistry through enzymes displays an astonishing degree of control. The legions of enzymes driving our metabolism facilitate thousands of chemical reactions at just the right time, in just the right place, and in an extraordinarily harmonized and measured manner with branching circuit boards of coordination. The catalysts facilitating our metabolism have all manner of built in controls: on/off switches, feedback loops, and subtle changes in their shape (called a conformational change) that slightly turn the dial that controls the rate of catalysis up or down.

How enzymes work to conduct our metabolism is through a gentle coercion—whispers of molecular manipulation. At the nanoscale of molecular biology everything operates by the interaction of positive and negative charges. These charges behave like the magnets you may have played with as a child. Put two positively charged ends together and the magnets push back, repelling each other. The same applies to the two negatively charged ends. But when a positively charged end and a negatively charged end are slid near each other they attract one another, gaining force until they snap loudly together. Like charges repel and opposites attract. These same, simple forces dominate all the molecular interactions occurring in the cell.

In chemistry, one of the central lessons is that every atom has a different affinity for electrons. This has an important consequence for cell biology: the surface of large molecules (like proteins) comprised of many different atoms has a richly diverse landscape of charge; positively and negatively charged nooks, valleys and hills exist across the topography of every large molecule's three-dimensional surface. This results in a mosh pit of interaction—an immense variety of molecules with differing charges are constantly repelling, attracting, twisting and pulling at one another within the cellular milieu. Each enzyme is imbued with something called an active site where the chemical reaction is facilitated.

Imagine an enzyme dedicated to breaking a long stick-like molecule in half. Now imagine the stick-like molecule has a slight positive charge on each end and a slight negative charge in the middle. To catalyze the reaction, the active site of the enzyme would be structurally opposite with respect to charge: having slight negative charges in locations corresponding to the ends of the stick-like molecule in order to attract it and firmly hold it within the active site. Now, imagine the active site to have a positive charge hovering at a location slightly above the negatively-charged center of the stick-like molecule. This will pull (because opposite charges attract) the middle of the stick-like molecule upward, bending it in the middle. The physical contortion of the now bent molecule stresses the bonds and "catalyzes" the breaking of it in half. This is how enzymes drive our metabolism, by manipulating, bending and contorting molecules in ways that subtly pressure them to react in a myriad different ways—breaking apart into new molecules, rearranging atoms within the molecule, or swapping atoms with nearby molecules to form new molecules—facilitating molecules that would not normally react into reacting.

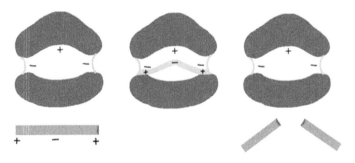

Illustration showing how a biological enzyme
catalyzes a chemical reaction

Even though Krebs had filled in the center of the metabolic map a conspicuous void remained. Krebs had linked the glycolytic pathway to the Krebs cycle, but then the map again went murky. The beginning (glycolysis) and the middle

(Krebs cycle) needed to be connected to the end (the cyto-chromes). Over "many years of patient work," using inhibi-tors in the same way Warburg used carbon monoxide to start and stop the reactions of the cytochromes, Keilin had proven that his original hypothesis about the cytochromes was correct: the cytochromes acted like a wire, with elec-trons traveling from one cytochrome to the next, reacting with oxygen at the final cytochrome in the chain, cyto-chrome a (now called cytochrome oxidase). But Keilin's concept of an *electron transport chain* left a critical question unanswered: How were the electrons fed into the begin-ning of the chain? Where did the electrons come from? Redox reactions, everyone knew, always occur in pairs. Warburg and Krebs had shown that the electron transport chain ended with a reduction, when electrons pass to oxy-gen thus reducing it, but the oxidation reaction, the *source* of the electrons for the electron transport chain, remained a mystery.

Ironically, it was Warburg—who initially disagreed with Keilin's suggestion of an electron transport chain—who provided the answer. In the late 1930s, Warburg isolated the compound in question. It was present in such vanishingly small quantities that Warburg needed 200 liters of horse blood to isolate a few milligrams. The compound Warburg discovered was a coenzyme called *nicotinamide adenosine dinucleotide,* or NAD+ for short—a compound composed of vitamin B3. NAD+ (critical to this story as we will see later) was the elusive source of electrons for the electron transport chain. Warburg's discovery of NAD+ provided the critical link between the glycolytic pathway, the Krebs cycle, and the electron transport chain. As glucose was broken down step-by-step, first in the glycolytic pathway and then the Krebs cycle, the electrons were stripped away and transferred to NAD+ and thus generating NADH (adding an electron to NAD+ makes NADH). NADH then acted as an intermediate, shuttling electrons to the beginning of the electron transport chain.

With the metabolic map becoming more and more complete, a gnawing question was still unanswered: How was energy *conserved*? When a candle burns, the energy is released as heat that quickly dissipates into the air, but energy metabolism in the body *requires* the energy to be captured in a usable form. *How* was it captured?

For biochemists in the 1930s this question was terribly daunting. Illuminating how the cell generated energy from food had proven remarkably complex: pathways, cycles, intermediates, electron transport chains. Yet this fundamental question remained unanswered. The first step toward solving it came from a German biochemist, Karl Lohman, who worked for Meyerhof. Lohmann stumbled on to a curious compound, *adenosine triphosphate*, ATP for short, that he isolated from liver and muscle tissue. Lohmann didn't know what role ATP played in the cell but in 1935, a Russian scientist named Vladimir

Engelhart, made the observation that ATP was required for muscles to contract. Engelhart's observation hinted that ATP might indeed be a carrier of energy. Then, a wandering Spanish-American scientist named Severo Ochoa made a critically important discovery: a single molecule of glucose fully processed through glycolysis, the Krebs cycle and the electron transport chain generated 38 molecules of ATP. Ochoa's experiments showed that the energy-producing pathways and ATP synthesis were somehow correlated. Even so, researchers at the time were skeptical that a single molecule could be the elusive carrier of cellular energy. Everyone assumed it *had* to be more complex.

But then an elegant frenzy of experiments performed between 1939 and 1941 by Fritz Lipmann—a Jewish scientist who also worked in Meyerhof's laboratory and fled Germany at the same time as Meyerhof— showed unequivocally that ATP was "the universal energy currency" of life—all life—from bacteria, amoebas and plants to reptiles, amphibians and mammals. The fact that all cellular energy production was conserved in a single molecule astonished investigators. And frankly, led to a collective sigh of relief. They had been climbing a mountain and the summit suddenly emerged from the fog. "It seems that in the field of biochemistry we have a rare example of progress leading to simplification," Lipmann would write.

When nature conserves a molecule or a metabolic pathway across the animal kingdom, it alludes to something deeper—something *so* mechanistically important that change is nonnegotiable—something protected from evolution's inexorable drive for variation. There may be many iterations of cars—color, shape, even type of motor, for example, but round wheels are conserved across all makes and models—they are essential to the functionality of a car. To look at an amoeba compared to a bird compared to a human, one would be forgiven for assuming the inner molecular mechanics were as different as the outside appearances. Yet it is not so. All life collapses to a handful of commonalities. Like DNA, like amino acids, like glycolysis and the Krebs cycle, ATP is shared by all life; it is the wheel to the car.

ATP is made from three components: the sugar ribose, three phosphate groups, and the nitrogenous base adenine (the same nitrogenous base used in DNA). ATP can be visualized as a core molecule with three phosphate groups dangling off the side. The usable energy in ATP is held in the bond between the second and the last phosphate group. When this bond is broken, ADP (adenosine diphosphate) is formed and a phosphate group is released. Here's the crux: ATP is chemically predisposed to turn into ADP + P, in the same way a ball perched on top of a hill is predisposed to roll down. ADP + P is much more stable than ATP—as is the ball once it comes to rest at the bottom of the hill. If you were to put some ATP in a test tube in the evening, by the morning almost all of it would have broken down into ADP + P. As such, ATP can be thought of as a charged battery, or as water hauled to the top of a waterfall. ATP is full of *potential energy*. Enzymes in the cell then *couple* themselves to ATP to power metabolic process. The same way a waterwheel *couples* itself to a waterfall to capture the energy of the falling water, or the way electronics are powered by *coupling* themselves to the energy in a charged battery. Our metabolism, by itself, sits lifeless. Yet, when ATP is added, our metabolism springs to life—DNA replicates, enzymes are manufactured, muscle contracts, immune cells fight off invaders and electrical impulses course through neurons.

When ATP is produced, it diffuses throughout the cell—like little batteries floating freely—providing power to every nook and cranny. And in that lies the genius in nature's design—funneling energy metabolism from many sources (foods) down to a single molecule that can be evenly distributed to power the cell's needs—like molecular Wi-Fi signaling, a ubiquitous source that all the users (enzymes) can tap into. ATP is what's known as a coenzyme. To power a metabolic reaction a coenzyme literally *partners* with enzymes. Consider muscle. Muscle consists of two fibers laid parallel next to each other: actin and myosin. Actin is like a rope; myosin is like a rope, too, but with arms that project out sequentially along the length of the fiber. To facilitate movement, ATP binds to the myosin arms and the high energy bond is broken, forming ADP and a negatively charged phosphate group. The interaction between the newly exposed negative charges repel and attract the positive and negative charges on the myosin arm, inducing a conformational change that causes the arm to grab the actin filament, yank it, then let go; like a person pulling a rope using one arm at a time.

ATP is central to metabolism—powering over a thousand known cellular reactions. ATP is the currency of cellular energy the same way money is the currency of an economy—having a single currency greatly simplifies the system. And just like the measure of turnover in monetary transactions measures the vibrancy of an economy, the degree of ATP's churn in the cell speaks to its central role in powering living organisms. At any given moment, the human body has about nine ounces of ATP diffused throughout its forty trillion cells—an unremarkable amount. It is the turnover that is remarkable. In a single day, your body churns though its own weight in ATP.

Back to the story. With the vital role of ATP now revealed by Lipmann, the next questions were obvious: *Where* was ATP made? Where, on the rapidly crystalizing metabolic map, did ATP synthesis lie? And perhaps more critically: *How* was ATP made? And thus began one of the most theatrical scientific dramas to ever take place.

ANTIESTABLISHMENT CHEMISTRY

The first example of ATP generation came from Efrin Racker, a Poland-born biochemist working in New York. Racker showed that glycolysis generates two ATP molecules by a process called *substrate-level phosphorylation*. As glucose was broken down in the glycolytic pathway, some of the energy from the chemical reactions was extracted and transferred to combine ADP with a phosphate group, thus forming ATP. As Racker showed, substrate-level phosphorylation is straightforward chemistry, the typical swapping and rearranging of atoms that enzymes facilitate. Like all known metabolic reactions, it requires physical interaction. The reactants—a metabolite of glucose, ADP, a phosphate group and the enzyme—must all come together in space and time for the reaction to take place. Yet Racker's substrate-level phosphorylation accounted for only 2 of the 38 ATP generated by respiration.

Finally, in 1948, the location of ATP synthesis was discovered by Albert Lehninger and Eugene Kennedy at Johns

Hopkins in Baltimore. Critically, they showed that the site of respiration was the tiny cellular organelles called mitochondria. Each cell contains roughly four hundred of the oval shaped structures of bacterial origin (mitochondria evolved from a free-living bacterium that was engulfed by another cell—they even retain a small circular genome as an icon of their former independence). Lehninger and Kennedy revealed mitochondria's unique structure: a smooth outer membrane surrounds a convoluted inner membrane and the space between the outer and inner membranes is called the inner-membrane space—and the central space defined by the inner membrane is called the matrix. The *inner membrane*, Lehninger and Kennedy showed, is saturated with the cytochromes. ATP was found to be *spilling* out of the mitochondria—and clearly the cytochromes were involved—but investigators had yet to show how electrons traveling from one cytochrome complex to the next—Keilin's electron transport chain—generate ATP.

In 1962, the unprecedented magnification and resolution of the newly developed electron microscope, revealed thousands and thousands of "mushroom shaped knobs" positioned alongside the cytochrome complexes within the *inner mitochondrial membrane*. It was suspected that these unusual structures had something to do with energy generation but no one was yet sure of their purpose. Then, in a "brilliant series of biological reconstitutions experiments," Racker showed the particles were in fact the enzyme responsible for generating ATP from ADP and phosphate. The enzyme, aptly named *ATP synthase*, was christened "The fundamental particles of biology." The focus now turned to ATP synthase. The critical question now was: *How* is ATP synthase generating ATP?

The limits of Racker's imagination were drawn from his previous experience with glycolysis. *To a man with a hammer, everything looks like a nail*—for Racker—and all the other chemists for that matter—all they had ever known was the traditional enzyme-facilitated chemistry of substrate-level phosphorylation; it was their *hammer*. Perhaps predictably, Racker set forth the hypothesis that ATP synthase *must* be generating ATP like those generated during glycolysis: by substrate-level phosphorylation.

But this hypothesis presented a conundrum: the cytochromes and ATP synthase were confined within the mitochondrial inner membrane, unanchored to anything—like thousands and thousands of beach balls randomly floating on a lake. For ATP to be generated by substrate-level phosphorylation, as Racker suspected, it would require the cytochromes to physically interact with ATP synthase—for them to be physically tethered together. For substrate-level phosphorylation to occur, the chemists knew, contact was *required*.

Racker and others then proposed a solution: an *intermediate* molecule. When the electrons move through the electron transport chain, they reasoned, the energy must be used to attach a phosphate group to an intermediate molecule that then freely diffused to the active site of ATP synthase where substrate-level phosphorylation could then take place—the phosphate group on the intermediate molecule could be transferred to ADP to form ATP. It was the *only* proposal that made sense. The hunt was on. The entire field hypnotically began searching for the hypothesized intermediate molecule.

But as one problem was solved another one surfaced. The production of ATP by substrate-level phosphorylation during glycolysis obeyed the rules of chemistry. One molecule of glucose generates 2 ATP and 2 molecules of pyruvate. Always. Chemists knew one thing for certain: chemical reactions balance—the numbers are whole and immutable. But when researchers attempted to reproduce the results of Ochoa's experiment that counted 38 ATPs formed per molecule of glucose respired, they kept getting different numbers. Sometimes 38 appeared, sometimes 36, sometimes 33—or any number in-between. The production of ATP by respiration, researchers realized, wasn't consistent and curiously seemed to skirt the uniform laws of chemical reactions.

As the hunt for the elusive intermediate continued yet another puzzling detail emerged: researchers discovered that respiration was dependent on an intact inner mitochondrial membrane. If it was disrupted in any way the generation of ATP within the mitochondria came to a screeching halt. Perhaps these curious observations should have prompted researchers to consider that ATP was being generated by an altogether different mechanism. Yet they didn't. Researchers, hobbled by their own imaginations, simply couldn't *conceive* of another way. There *had* to be an intermediate. For years the search went on. A decade passed. The metabolic map had hit the equivalent of the end of the world: an impassable void. One observer commented that the field had reached a state "little short of a crisis."

This was the state of the field of bioenergetics when a man named Peter Mitchell entered graduate school at Cambridge. Mitchell was not the typical graduate student of the 1940's—he styled his shoulder-length hair in the fashion of Beethoven, and wore bright-colored pants and a burgundy-purple blazer over a shirt unbuttoned all the way to his waist. He had an impish, youthful face that accentuated his unusual sense of humor. He had many interests apart from science: he loved music and the visual arts, agriculture, architecture and nature. Mitchell seemed to prefer the role of an outsider. Instead of eating in the dining hall or at one of the pubs frequented by other scientists, such as the Eagle (where Francis Crick would announce the discovery of the structure of DNA nearly a decade later), he felt more comfortable at the Peacock—a small diner run by a Jewish Czechoslovakian refugee, and frequented by foreigners, artists and musicians.

If one were to describe the scientific establishment at the time, rigid, wooden and evidence-based to a fault might come to mind. This was in sharp contrast to the era of Lavoisier, when theories with no falsifiability such as vitalism were freely proposed and freely accepted by even the most prominent scientists. Lavoisier could have been considered "anti-establishment" in the sense that his work was sharply more evidence-based than the prevailing scientific environment at the time. By Mitchell's era, though, the pendulum had swung in the opposite direction, and perhaps it had swung too far. The establishment discouraged, scorned and ridiculed conjecture beyond what the data unequivocally evidenced. This created a scientific culture that loathed inspired leaps of imagination without evidence to support them. Given this backdrop, Mitchell was fortunate to have been accepted into graduate school at Cambridge.

The department head, Sir Frederick Gowland Hopkins (he recruited Krebs as he fled Germany) had a reputation of having "a capacity to suffer fools gladly." One evening, at a party arranged for the biochemistry department, Mitchell and David Keilin (Keilin was also at Cambridge) happened upon each other at the hors d'oeuvre table. Keilin, eating olives, looked at Mitchell mischievously, and then flicked an olive into the crowd. To Mitchell, the act signaled defiance to the established way of thinking. "I was not accustomed to a professor behaving that way, so I was absolutely delighted. He maybe even did it because he knew I was an outsider and would be pleased, wishing I could do it myself." Keilin, too, could have been considered an "antiestablishment" scientist in that he was perfectly willing to propose theories based on imagination. After his discovery of cytochromes, he championed the idea of the electron transport chain before any evidence to support it existed. Warburg, a more traditional, establishment-type scientist, refused to acknowledge the existence of the electron transport chain until the evidence was irrefutable. If Keilin could be considered an antiestablishment thinker with his willingness to propose theoretical ideas, then Mitchell was definitely so. For Mitchell, science *began* with the imagination and then followed with experimental data. Mitchell preferred to let his imagination run free, to construct mental models of cells, organelles, and molecular interactions.

At Cambridge, Mitchell got away with his unconventional approach. But barely. His first thesis was rejected by the committee for "lacking empirical data." Keilin, who was angry that Mitchell's thesis was rejected, remarked "Peter is too original for his examiners." To be sure, Mitchell's research could be sloppy. Once, when Mitchell was giving a presentation on his research, Hans Krebs was heard mumbling, "but he hasn't done the controls." But his "lack of controls" were, metaphorically, the wellspring from which his genius flowed, eschewing any shackles of tradition. It was a fair trade: in return, he had the gift of a wandering mind. In many professions a wandering mind is a liability, but for a scientist it could be a virtue. Indeed, perhaps one of the greatest scientists of the era, Albert Einstein, was notorious for wandering aimlessly outside or riding his bike in circles while his imagination reached to the stars. "Creativity is the residue of time wasted," he once quipped.

Eventually Mitchell found even the loose structure at Cambridge too confining. He accepted an invitation to set up his own bioenergetics unit at the University of Edinburgh where, he felt, a less restrictive climate prevailed. The field of bioenergetics was still at a standstill, held captive by the dogmatic assumption that to generate ATP, ATPase had to react with an elusive intermediate molecule. But the collective search had yet to find it.

By 1960, Mitchell decided to focus more intensely on the problem. He had a hunch. He had done previous work on bacteria and his imagination wandered between the two. Specifically, he studied a process called *active transport*—cellular machinery used to acquire the molecules a bacterium needed, or conversely, to expel unwanted molecules. Active transport, as the name implies, requires energy. It is accomplished by protein pumps that expend ATP energy to pump molecules into or out of the cell.

Using his vibrant imagination, Mitchell extended the functionality of these protein pumps further. He imagined protein pumps that pumped atoms into a confined space, increasing the concentration, like air being pumped into an air compressor. Once full, an air compressor has stored energy. The energy from the confined air can then be captured to power pneumatic tools. The same concept would hold true in the cell, he imagined. He began jotting his ideas down in a notebook.

By 1961, Mitchell's hypothesis was complete, and he decided to unveil it to the world. In its complete form, it looked like this: food is eaten and digested into its component parts: fats, amino acids and carbohydrates are broken down and eventually processed through the Krebs cycle, releasing carbon dioxide and generating NADH. NADH then feeds electrons into the starting point of the electron transport chain leaving behind NAD+ that is regenerated back to NADH in the Krebs cycle. The electrons are then passed from one cytochrome complex to the next, like electrons moving through a wire (pulled by electron-hungry oxygen at the end of the line), until they reach Warburg's cytochrome oxidase where they are combined with oxygen and protons to form water. But here's the key: the cytochrome complexes, rather than capturing the energy of the flowing electrons to generate the still-undiscovered intermediate, according to Mitchell, used the energy to pump protons from the matrix of the mitochondria into the intermembrane space. As such, the intermembrane space becomes filled up with protons like the reservoir of an air compressor. Now, claimed Mitchell, the pressure generated from a confined space filled with positively charged protons, is endowed with potential energy from both a concentration gradient and an electrical gradient. This energy, reasoned Mitchell, could then be harnessed. Recall that ATPase, the enzyme known to generate ATP, floats within the two-dimensional space of the inner-mitochondrial membrane—like beach balls on a lake. In truth, ATPase spans across the membrane, so it is better imagined like cocktail straws poking through a taut piece of plastic wrap. All this built up to the pièce de résistance of Mitchell's new hypothesis: as the pent-up protons flow back across the membrane, through ATPase, the energy from the flow of protons is used to transfer a phosphate group onto ADP, thus forming ATP (similar to how pneumatic tools are powered by the flow of air). The generation of ATP, said Mitchell, is due to what he called *chemiosmotic coupling*: chemo, denoting the chemical gradient formed by the protons and osmotic from the Greek *to push*.

When Mitchell's new chemiosmotic theory was published in the esteemed journal *Nature,* it was instantly met with ridicule, scorn, or worse—it was outright ignored. There were two interesting and opposing elements to Mitchell's idea. First—not unusual for Mitchell—he proposed it as a raw theory, without *any* experimental data to back it up. "There wasn't a shred of evidence in its favor," commented a colleague. But intriguingly, if one looked carefully, it was apparent that Mitchell's theory solved all the questions plaguing ATP formation. Number one, it explained why an intact membrane was necessary. And number two, it explained how an uneven number of ATP could be generated per electron flowing through the electron transport chain; since the process didn't occur in a one-to-one chemical interaction, some inefficiency was sure to occur as protons were able to leak across the membrane on occasion, by-passing ATP synthase. Even so, the establishment, as a whole, thought Mitchell's theory was laughable. Racker, who was one of a handful willing to consider that Mitchell's theory might be right, gently professed, "Peter's ideas have not been treated too kindly by the investigators in the field."

Mitchell's theory was a radical rethink of an existing scientific paradigm. If history is a guide, the architects of transformative ideas are in for a dust-up. Galileo was almost killed for his heretical new image of the solar system; Einstein almost lost his position for his bohemian suggestion that everything is relative and nothing is absolute. For the next fifteen years, Mitchell would defend his theory against wave after wave of attacks. For the field of bioenergetics, the contentious period came to be known as the "ox phos wars" (short for oxidative phosphorylation). The war was largely played out in the journals but also erupted at a yearly conference dedicated to ox phos research. These annual meetings often became heated, combative and highly personal. "The oxidative phosphorylation field had the reputation that if you went to a Federation meeting, all the meetings were crowded because everybody went along because they knew there would be a damned good fight there," said a contemporary observer. Cancer researcher, Young Ko, received her PhD under Peter Pedersen at Johns Hopkins, who received his degree under Albert Lehninger, also at Hopkins. Lehninger, Pedersen and Ko were among a handful of researchers who believed in Mitchell's theory. During those years Pederson spent a lot of time counselling Peter Mitchell on his visits to the United States. Mitchell would come into Pedersen's office and Peter would encourage them to carry on. "They were terribly depressed. Pete would say, 'Someday the world will know you are right.' You have to remember the field of bioenergetics was *huge* back then. And the controversy surrounding Mitchell's theory was fierce. There was hate involved," said Ko.

Normally a warm, gregarious person, Mitchell felt compelled to aggressively fight back. Ultimately, he began to question human nature and people's intentions. "On the one hand, he deplored the failure of his colleagues to proceed by cool rational argument and their tendency to personalize situations, a position that caused him to think hard and deep about the nature of communication between scientists and between humans generally," wrote his biographer. As the years passed, the fight took a personal toll on Mitchell. He left the University of Edinburgh and retreated to a personal laboratory he had constructed from an abandoned house in Cornwall. His health, already bad, became worse.

You may wonder, and rightfully so, how could a scientific debate last for 15 years? The answer is simple: biology is a messy affair. Biology is not like physics where a single, clean experiment can be definitive. Figuring out what is happening in the nanoscale environment of a cell full of thousands of different compounds is a difficult task under even the best experimental conditions. To conclude that a theory is correct is often decided by totality of evidence, and this takes time.

By the mid-1970s, the totality of evidence began to accumulate in favor of Mitchell's theory. The attacks came less and less frequently. The few remaining detractors began to be the outsiders. And then in 1978 Mitchell received a call. It was the Nobel committee informing him that he had won the Nobel Prize for his contribution to bioenergetics. In his Nobel acceptance speech, Mitchell began with the battle—and the revenge—which had dominated a good chunk of his life. "It was obviously my hope that the chemiosmotic [theory] might one day come to be generally accepted, and I have done my best to argue in favor of that state of affairs for more than twenty years . . . was it not the great Max Planck who remarked that a new scientific idea does not triumph by convincing its opponents, but rather because its opponents eventually die? The fact that what began as the chemiosmotic hypothesis has now been acclaimed as the chemiosmotic theory . . . has therefore aroused in me emotions of astonishment and delight in full and equal measure, which are all the more heartfelt because those who were formerly my most capable opponents are still in the prime of their scientific lives." Mitchell may have been largely vindicated, yet even after his Nobel Prize remnants of the ox phos war still smoldered, a prominent biochemist said that Mitchell received the Nobel Prize for "bioimagination."

With Mitchell's triumph, the metabolic map was now complete. Lavoisier's distant dream of understanding the flame of life was finally realized. It was a marriage of the traditional with new and exotic chemistry: beautifully evolved enzymes bend, twist and pull the molecules from the *three known sources of food* (protein, carbohydrate and fats) through a series of rearrangements and then through a merry-go-round process of electron extraction. The electrons are then handed off to complex I, now known to be comprised of proteins in addition to the iron-containing cytochrome. Electrons are then shuttled to complex III and IV by the nimbler intermediates Coenzyme Q and Cytochrome C. Each time an electron passes through an electron transport chain complex a proton is pumped into the intermembrane space, creating an electrical and chemical gradient. And finally, ATP is generated by ATPase, a nanoscale marvel of engineering powered like a hydroelectric dam from the steady flow of protons down the chemiosmotic gradient back into the mitochondrial matrix.

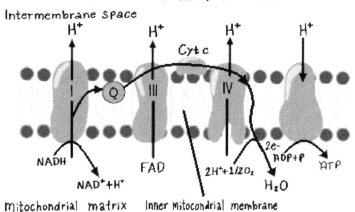

Illustration of the Electron Transport Chain
as elucidated by Peter Mitchell

With Mitchell's completion of the metabolic map, researchers went on to uncover the intricate and exquisite mechanisms that control human metabolism. Tight feed-back loops ensure that only the needed amount of fuel is burned. Yet, they showed metabolism is also remarkably flexible—geared to meet the needs arising from different circumstances. Under normal conditions, as you sit and read this book, your metabolism idles at a rate known as your *basal* metabolism, with just enough fuel flowing down the glycolytic pathway, into the Krebs cycle, then feed-ing the electron transport chain to generate exactly the amount of ATP needed to keep all your cellular processes operating efficiently. But imagine you set the book down, walk outside and encounter a swarm of angry bees. You run as fast as you can to get away. Your muscles go from needing 0.01 micromoles of ATP per second to approxi-mately 5 micromoles of ATP per second, a 50,000 percent increase. As you run, your aerobic pathways—Krebs cycle and the electron transport chain—are quickly maxed out. Electrons are transferred down the wire from carrier to carrier at a rate of about 1 electron every 5 to 20 millisec-onds. The Krebs cycle and the electron transport chain are capable of producing more ATP but are limited by the amount of oxygen that hemoglobin can carry—this is the *rate limiting step* for oxidative phosphorylation (that's why professional cyclists "blood dope" by injecting blood or a drug called EPO to make more hemoglobin). With demand greatly exceeding capacity, you need another way to generate ATP. Luckily for you, the glycolytic pathway has evolved to accommodate short bursts of energy. The glycolytic pathway has the excess enzymes needed to meet the demand for a massive and instantaneous increase in ATP production; like a fire department, the extra enzymes are always there *just in case* they are needed. The flux of glucose down the glycolytic pathway goes from a trickle to a torrent, flowing so fast that it quickly overwhelms the Krebs cycle's ability to process it. The end product, pyruvate, builds up quickly, piling up into a sort-of molecular dam capable of hindering the massive flow of glucose. Another enzyme leaps into action with the sole purpose of mopping up the excess pyruvate so the waterfall of glucose can continue to flow. This enzyme, lactate dehydrogenase, quickly converts pyruvate into lactate that then diffuses out of the cell through special transport proteins called monocarboxylic transport proteins.

You escaped the angry swarm of bees, but you injured your ankle while running. Back at home, lying on your couch after a large meal, you reset back to basal metabolism. Now, however, as fuel molecules flow through the metabolic map more of the metabolites are pulled out to enter the biosynthetic (anabolic) pathways necessary to repair your injury and return your body to homeostasis. The stem cells near your injury spring to life. As they begin to copy their DNA in preparation to divide and heal the damage, metabolites are pulled from the glycolytic pathway producing the nucleic acids needed to manufacture DNA. The oxidative stress you endured while running generated free radicals wreaking havoc within the cell. This requires the manufacture of more antioxidants to neutralize the free radicals. Metabolites are pulled from both the glycolytic pathway and Krebs cycle and processed through a series of reactions generating glutathione, the cell's "master" antioxidant. Energy-producing metabolism is the fountainhead of the living. It supplies the energy of movement to run from predators, to chase down prey, plow fields, and build civilizations. It also supplies the energy and building blocks of growth and renewal, healing and regeneration.

By the time researchers had a complete image of energy metabolism, in the 1970s, biology was in the throes of a new revolution. Watson and Crick unveiled the structure of DNA to the world in 1953. "We have discovered the secret of life!" Crick announced to the patrons of the Eagle Pub in the winter of 1953. The double helix immediately captivated the imaginations of a generation of biologists. Science, at no time before, or since, had the revelation of a molecular structure so utterly overflowing with implications; so enormously suggestive. Once the article announcing the discovery was circulated a line through history was drawn—a new era of molecular biology was born. "Images crystallize ideas—and the image of a double-helical molecule that carried the instructions to build, run, repair, and reproduce humans crystallized the optimism and wonder of the 1950s. Encoded in that molecule were the loci of human perfectibility and vulnerability: once we learned to manipulate this chemical, we would rewrite our nature. Diseases would be cured, fates changed, futures reconfigured," wrote a researcher. Laboratories, resources and imaginations stampeded from bioenergetics to genetics in hopes being part of "reconfiguring the future." Bioenergetics, the once-dominant field in biology, was cast aside—perceived as the musty old basement of biology—a relic of the past.

Yet, unknown to everyone, the map was not yet complete. There was one more fuel—the *fourth fuel*— that still needed its place on the map.

THE "GREAT" CONTROLLING
NUCLEOTIDE COENZYMES

I n the summer of 1966, while the ox phos war raged
on, Richard Veech, boarded the red-eye flight from
Washington, DC, to London on his way to the laboratory of Hans Krebs at Oxford University (Krebs moved
from the University of Sheffield to Oxford in 1954, one
year after winning the Nobel Prize). Veech had graduated from Harvard medical school one year earlier and
accepted a position as a physician for the NIH at St.
Elizabeth's Hospital in Washington, DC. While making
clinical rounds one evening Veech experienced the same
uncomfortable realization that both Krebs and Warburg
had as young doctors entering clinical medicine: "Well,
if you have been an intern and resident and you've seen a
few people die, you realize that you really don't know very
much at all. You better go learn some more. That's what I
did," said Veech. All three had an acute visceral awareness
of the massive chasm of knowledge that stood between the

basic science of disease and the practice of clinical medicine. With this realization, all three had experienced a life-changing moment of clarity; and all three decided, in that moment of clarity, to do something about it. Warburg, Krebs, and now Veech all made the decision to step away from the practice of medicine, shifting their efforts to understanding the fundamental processes underlying the diseases they were expected to treat.

Veech landed at Heathrow on a sweltering morning in early July, grabbed his luggage and boarded the train for the hour-long trip to Oxford. Indeed, it was highly unusual for a freshly minted medical doctor with very little laboratory training to have received an invitation to the now-famous laboratory of Sir Hans Krebs. Krebs was not in the business of training young students; he had accepted only 20 PhD students during his 50 years in research. At this stage of his career, the most distinguished scientists fought to work with Krebs; all the research positions in his laboratory were now filled exclusively by distinguished U.S. professors on sabbatical. Veech had been lucky. At the NIH he became friends with a physician turned biochemist, Han Weil Malherbe, who had served with Krebs in Freiburg. One evening, while listening to Veech lament about his new-found desire to learn biochemistry, Weil-Malherbe was moved to approach Krebs, convincing him to offer Veech a coveted position in his lab.

Veech arrived at Oxford at 9:00 a.m. As he juggled his unruly baggage and a map of the Oxford campus, he made his way to Krebs famous Metabolic Research

Laboratory—a sprawling bridge between two buildings, with a driveway beneath. Surprisingly, he was greeted by Krebs himself. Krebs was in an unusually energetic mood. He had just returned from a conference in the United States and was infused with a new found enthusiasm. Krebs had shifted the focus of his laboratory to a branch of metabolism that now fascinated him: *coenzymes*. Fritz Lipmann's earlier discovery—that all the branching complexities of energy metabolism funneled into ATP as a carrier of energy—hinted of a deeper order to bioenergetic metabolism. With ATP, the metabolic map collapsed to a "master regulator" of metabolism. With its ability to store energy and then diffuse throughout the cell, the energy balance of ATP alone dictated the fate of over a thousand metabolic reactions. Krebs's current fascination was the realization that there were other coenzymes in addition to ATP that also acted as master regulators. NAD+ and NADP+, like ATP, also drove massive swaths of the metabolic map. Warburg had discovered that NAD+ shuttles electrons to the beginning of the electron transport chain, but now, it was dawning on Krebs that NADH and NADPH had a broader purpose: to act like the universal carrier of energy ATP, and diffuse throughout the cell, acting like tiny batteries that power a myriad of other pivotal metabolic reactions.

Shortly after Warburg's discovery of NAD+, Fritz Lipmann discovered another critically important coenzyme—given the simple name *coenzyme A*. Coenzyme A is naturally synthesized in the cell from pantothenate (vitamin B5). Lipmann showed that coenzyme A was involved in an important step at the end of the glycolytic pathway that Krebs had missed: pyruvate → acetyl-CoA. (This didn't diminish Krebs's original unveiling of the Krebs cycle; additional intermediate reactions were often missed in those days simply due to limitations in the available technology.)

Lipmann showed that acetyl-CoA is the primary metabolite feeding into the Krebs cycle. Acetyl-CoA acts as a critically important hub on the metabolic map. It is the final product of *all* energy metabolism; carbohydrate, amino acids, and fats are all broken down into acetyl-CoA. As such, acetyl-CoA is more than just a metabolite feeding the Krebs cycle—it also acts like the other coenzymes; ATP, NADH and NADPH—a carrier of energy that drives a broad swath of metabolic reactions.

The importance of ATP as a carrier of energy was well established. But what Krebs now realized was that energy was also conserved within the other three coenzymes: NADH, NADPH and acetyl-CoA. Like ATP, these three coenzymes capture energy to power the metabolic reactions that occur in all the various cellular compartments: the nucleus, mitochondria, and cytoplasm. Each coenzyme operates as a *couple*, meaning it has a high energy form and a low energy form. ATP is the high energy form and ADP is the low energy form. Like ATP, the other three coenzymes act like tiny batteries that are charged by the combustion engine at the heart of metabolism: glycolysis Krebs cycle   electron transport chain. Just like a battery, the degree of "charge" can be measured by the ratio of the high energy form to the low energy form. In the case of ATP, for example, more ATP relative to ADP correlates to a more "charged" battery. Same with the ratio of NADH to NAD+ and NADPH to NADP+ and Acetyl CoA to CoA. Once charged, the coenzymes then run our metabolism: diffusing throughout the cell, powering the thousands of reactions that occur moment to moment.

At the conference, Veech's former professor at Harvard, George Cahill, had asked Krebs what the ratio of NADPH to NADP+ was. In other words, how charged was the NADP+ couple's battery? Krebs confessed he did not know. For that matter, nobody knew. In that moment, Krebs realized that this was critical to a holistic understanding of metabolism due to his growing realization that the four coenzyme couples were powering virtually *every* metabolic reaction.

The importance of these four coenzymes to the entirety of human metabolism was on Krebs's mind as Veech walked into his laboratory. Veech barely had time to set his bags down before Krebs hurried him into his office (which more closely resembled a doorless closet). Krebs excitedly informed Veech that his first project was to determine the ratio of NADPH to NADP+ within the cytoplasm. He then introduced Veech to the scientist who would train him, fellow Harvard graduate Pat Lund. There was an awkward pause. Veech realized that Krebs expected him to leave his bags in the corner and begin his training now. Exhausted, Veech sheepishly explained that he was scheduled to procure his lodging and unpack, but would be ready to start first thing in the morning.

The next morning, Veech, still jet lagged, showed up at Krebs's laboratory early. Like Warburg, Krebs ran a tight ship. Work was expected to begin at 9 a.m. sharp. Veech was starting from scratch. Pat Lund, a steady hand for Krebs over the years, began with the basics, starting with the proper technique to measure the metabolites from known metabolic reactions occurring within the cell. To do this, they used *freeze clamped liver*: a slice of liver tissue flash frozen to stop the entirety of cellular metabolism at once. It provided a snapshot of metabolic activity in the actual milieu of the cell. It was like freezing New York City to measure economic activity. One could then count the number of cars on the streets, people in museums, restaurants and offices to determine the state of the economy at a given moment in time.

It was too technically challenging to measure the ratio of the coenzymes directly. It had to be done indirectly, the same way Krebs and Warburg had co-opted the properties of carbon dioxide to indirectly determine which of the cytochromes was reacting with oxygen. Because the coenzymes powered the vast majority of metabolic reactions, they could simply measure the ratio of the reactants to products of a metabolic reaction powered by a given coenzyme, that, in turn, would reveal the ratio of the coenzyme itself. Imagine it this way: you're trying to determine the voltage (energy) within a transmission line. But you can't measure it directly. Instead, you measure the power output of an electrical device connected to the transmission line. By measuring the metabolic reactions powered by the coenzymes Veech could reveal the energy within the coenzyme couple itself.

In only a few months, Veech was proficient enough in basic bench chemistry and was largely left alone. He immediately realized a glaring mistake made by other laboratories doing similar research. Specifically, the other labs were grinding up the entire cell then measuring the metabolic reactions linked to the coenzymes. This experimental approach, Veech realized, did not capture the true ratio of the coenzymes. The reason: the ratios of the coenzymes were *very* different in each of the different cellular compartments. The cytoplasm, for example, has different metabolic needs than those of the mitochondria and the nucleus, and therefore houses differently charged coenzymes. Each coenzyme couple in each cellular compartment, Veech realized, would require separate measurement. To determine the ratio of the cytoplasmic NADP+ couple—the task assigned to him—Veech searched for the metabolic reactions powered by the NADP+ coenzyme that occurred *exclusively* in the cytoplasm, and focused on those. How far the reaction was driven to completion (the ratio of reactant to products) would reveal the energy of the cytoplasmic NADP+ couple. A more complete reaction (more products relative to reactants) corresponded to a more powerfully "charged" NADPH to NADP+ ratio. A less complete reaction (more reactants relative to products) would correspond to a less "charged" NADPH coenzyme couple.

As the weeks turned to months and the months rolled into a year, Veech found the work in Krebs laboratory deeply meaningful. What Veech was revealing was the stunning beauty of the universe at its most interesting: *life*. Einstein had revealed a beautifully woven tapestry of laws that stitched the present to the past. Now Veech's research, too, was revealing an interwoven tapestry that transcended time. All four nucleotide coenzymes were built from a simple precursor: adenosine monophosphate. This commonality adumbrated an ancient and critically important functionality—a cornerstone that evolution could build on as the free energy from the sun was spun to new heights of complexity.

His relationship with Krebs had also grown and was a source of deep satisfaction for Veech. "He loved Krebs," said one of Veech's closest friends. "Krebs loved him, too. He was his guy." Like the commonality of the nucleotide coenzymes they were researching, there was an underlying commonality to Krebs's and Veech's careers. Krebs wouldn't be where he was without luck. Warburg had taken a chance with Krebs on the recommendation of a friend. Krebs, too, had taken a chance with Veech, also on the recommendation of a friend. He could have easily given his spot to any one of a number of distinguished professors on his waiting list. Perhaps, on some level, he felt he was paying it forward. "He considered his training with Warburg crucial. In his autobiography . . . Krebs wrote 'Among all my teachers, he had by far the greatest influence on my development and I owe him an immense debt.' Many who worked with Hans Krebs, including myself, would say the same of him," wrote Veech.

By the Christmas of 1967, Veech had accomplished the original project Krebs had assigned to him: determining the ratio of cytoplasmic NADPH to NADP. He had also accomplished something larger. Krebs had been quick to recognize the importance of the four nucleotide coenzymes to the *entirety* of metabolism, but Veech's research revealed something deeper: a surprising expanse of entwined relationships—a metabolic ecosystem that had not been fully appreciated. To read a biochemistry textbook is page after page of separate metabolic pathways—cholesterol synthesis, hormone synthesis, urea formation, energy metabolism, and so on. The student comes away with the image that each process operates independent of the other. The textbooks paint a picture of metabolism as the sum of a vast collection of loosely associated pathways. What Veech presented to Krebs that Christmas break was a different picture of metabolism—one that lay bare an internal harmony—an image of metabolic networks stitched together into a unified field.

This metabolic interconnectedness emanates from the internal design: the vast majority of the thousands of reactions that comprise human metabolism are powered by the four nucleotide coenzymes. They are continuously charged by the food we eat and the air we breathe and then diffuse throughout our cells to power our metabolism. Veech showed that even the nucleotide coenzymes do not operate independently—they, too, are linked together. The cytoplasmic NAD+ couple is linked to the cytoplasmic ATP couple, which is linked to the mitochondrial NAD+ couple, which is linked to the mitochondrial ATP couple, which is linked to the mitochondrial NADPH couple, which is linked to the cytoplasmic NADP+ couple, and so on and so on. Our metabolism was not a series of independent pathways as conveyed by the textbooks; instead, it was an intertwined network of reactions—an ecology—with the four nucleotide coenzymes working as hubs in the center. The implications of this realization with regard to fundamental health were profound. Why? Because a change in energy of one coenzyme couple rippled through the system affecting the other coenzyme couples and from there vast swaths of the metabolic map. If the energy in the mitochondrial NAD+ coenzyme was reduced, for example, so was the energy of ATP, and the over a thousand reactions coupled to ATP. Implicit in Veech's research was the realization that if energy metabolism was diminished, or slowed in any way, virtually every biological process would suffer. Conversely, if there was a way to boost the charge of the coenzyme couples, the entirety of metabolism would become more efficient, "supercharged," *so to speak*. Energy production, detoxification pathways, the neurotransmitter production that colors our mood and emotion . . . everything would simply *work better*. Yet Veech knew of no way to do this . . . *for now*.

Approximate number of metabolic reactions powered by each of the Nucleotide Coenzymes

ATP = 1084

NADPH = 90

NADH = 98

Acetyl CoA = 226

From Veech's publication describing the above figure: "The relative numbers of enzyme-linked reactions in which the controlling nucleotide couples are reactants and products."

Veech RL;Todd King M;Pawlosky R;Kashiwaya Y;Bradshaw PC;Curtis W; "The 'Great' Controlling Nucleotide Coenzymes." IUBMB Life, U.S. National Library of Medicine.

At first glance, Krebs was incredulous of the data Veech presented to him. "That can't be right," said Krebs. "Well damn it, it is," Veech shot back. Of the moment, Veech would later write, "Neither of us were angry, we were just expressing our opinions freely, which was both of our habits. Krebs never became out of sorts when discussing experiments, even if they were critical, only when people, often visiting professors, wanted to talk, and waste his time."

Krebs walked away without saying a word. He didn't bring up Veech's research for the next month. It was clear to Veech that Krebs was, in his own way, mulling over the implications in his mind. He then approached Veech and simply stated that it was time to write the paper. In the end, it was the longest paper of Krebs's career and one of the few publications he deemed "his most important."

THE HERO

In the fall of 1968, Veech had completed most of the work needed for his doctoral thesis. He was scheduled to present his research at a conference in Boston that October. After the conference—and before returning to Oxford to wrap up his final project—he decided to visit a cousin in Hanover, New Hampshire. It was raining in Boston as the Northeast Airlines twin-engine jet prop took off. After an hour of uneventful cruising, the captain announced he was starting the final approach into the Hanover airport. Veech looked out the window. In between blankets of thick fog, an occasional sliver of land appeared. The ground appeared uncomfortably close. He then heard an abrupt snapping sound. There was an eerie moment of silence and a twisting motion that felt very wrong. Next, a sudden piercing noise and a flash of light as he was slammed forward into the seat in front of him. Clumps of mud flew into his face, blinding him for a moment. And then silence. It took a moment for what had just happened to register. Due to the heavy fog and a faulty altitude reading sent from the airport, the airplane, upon descent, had crashed into the rocky and heavily wooded peak of Moose Mountain, sixty feet below its summit. There were 42 people on board the plane.

Veech gathered himself. The acrid scent of foreign materials burning filled the air. He noticed a crack in the fuselage and clawed his way toward it. He was able to shimmy through the gap and escape the wreckage. He could now see what had happened. The airplane was broken into two pieces. The front was half buried into the side of the mountain and engulfed in flames. Bodies, luggage, airplane parts and tree limbs were illuminated by the fire. None of the thirty-two in front survived. The nine passengers and one stewardess in the back of the plane had survived the crash, but many were badly injured. Veech set about tending to the injured as best he could. He then heard screaming from the wreckage. Veech tried to convince others to help him go free the person but most were too scared or injured. Finally, Robert Kimball, an assistant dean at Dartmouth, agreed to help and the two rushed back into the wreckage. He "marshalled us all . . . and got us going," said Kimball. They reached the pinned man and began clearing the wreckage to free him. The clock was ticking. They could smell fuel and even see it dripping from the debris. Pieces of fabric were burning throughout the wreckage. The man begged not to move him, crying out in pain but Veech and Kimball disregarded his pleas and pulled him from the debris. Seconds after they got him to a safe distance, the remains ignited into an intense blaze, engulfing all that remained. After interviewing the survivors, the local newspaper declared Veech "the real hero" of the incident, risking his own life to save another, and doing so despite the injuries he had suffered: a crushed vertebra, broken rib and multiple lacerations on his head and face.

A few hours later the rescue crew arrived and hauled the survivors down the mountain on stretchers. Veech was taken to the Mary Hitchcock Memorial Hospital in Hanover. Otto Warburg, once asked about his time serving on the front lines in World War I, said, "I was taught that one must be more than one appears to be." That night on Moose Mountain, Veech was much more than he appeared to be.

After healing from his injuries, Veech moved his family back to the United States and began looking for a job. He eventually took a position at the NIH, this time, not as a doctor but as a researcher, where he would pick up where he had left off in Oxford. The metabolic consequences of the interconnectedness of the nucleotide coenzymes still captivated his attention. Life, by definition, is a battle against *equilibrium*. To reach equilibrium is to go from order to chaos, when all of an organism's highly structured macromolecules dissolve and scatter into their most elementary state. The moment we enter the world we are thrust in an incessant battle with entropy. Our bodies are like a handful of marbles held by a hand that grows increasingly frail, eventually losing its grip and dropping them to scatter into a final equilibrium. Every moment of our lives our metabolism fights the good fight against equilibrium by "charging" the nucleotide coenzymes into a more energetic state. They, then, use the energy infused in them to push back against other metabolic equilibriums to maintain order. Energy metabolism's biggest task—the front line in the battle—is the maintenance of inorganic ion gradients between the interior and exterior of the cell. Every animal cell membrane is saturated in nanoscale protein pumps that pump out three sodium ions while simultaneously allowing two potassium ions to enter the cell. Each pump cycle spends the energy of one ATP. Maintaining this critical equilibrium between sodium and potassium is expensive, costing roughly 30 percent of the ATP we generate. For nerve cells the cost is higher, roughly 70 percent of ATP. The gradient of sodium and potassium in turn powers many other cellular processes: the firing of neurons, transporting nutrients like glucose and amino acids into the cell, and controlling cell volume. Veech spent the next decade at the NIH researching this vastly entangled relationship between inorganic ions and the nucleotide coenzyme system.

One of the requirements for maintaining a lab at the NIH was an annual review where colleagues within a field of study were invited to personally review the lab in question. Veech's annual reviews looked more like a VIP gathering than a typical NIH review. Krebs made the trip to Veech's lab every year until his death in 1981. The great Albert Lehninger often came, as did an elite list of other distinguished scientists. "These were the most enjoyable and stimulating meetings I have ever been privileged to attend. The reviewers received the grand sum of $75 per day, over a 2-day weekend, and a free dinner at a cheap restaurant funded by the laboratory chief since government rules prevent such amenities as free food. Nonetheless, they appeared to enjoy these meetings as much as the laboratory staff and students," Veech would later write.

During the 1980s, Veech sensed that the atmosphere at the NIH had begun to change. "By the mid-1980s, review processes at NIH became more bureaucratized . . . The work of our laboratory went from being a 'national treasure' to a 'waste of money,' depending upon the eye of the beholder. By 1991, our work at NIH was judged to be inadequate, and I was notified that the laboratory would be shut down in 2 years' time."

Faced with losing his laboratory at the NIH, Veech had to make a decision. He had two years to change the minds of the reviewers. By now he had shifted away from the biochemistry of inorganic ions and had become intensely interested in *ketone metabolism*, an obscure and marginally studied shift to a metabolic state that occurs during periods of starvation, or when a person deliberately fasts or when the intake of carbohydrates is drastically reduced—favoring fats in its place, referred to as a "ketogenic diet." He had been introduced to ketone metabolism by his former professor at Harvard, George Cahill. To his surprise, his staff agreed to stay, even though it appeared that the ship was sinking. "To their great credit, the laboratory members, who were all to be terminated at the end of this period, accepted my explanation that this was a 'Birkenhead drill' and stayed at their posts, completing the work outlined during the remaining 2 years," said Veech. They had two years. He was betting *everything* on ketones.

THE FOURTH FUEL

I n the early 1990s, few had heard of ketone metabolism. George Cahill was one of maybe two or three
biochemists who were actively studying these obscure
molecules. Cahill was aware of the strange history of
ketones. Ketone metabolism was intimately connected
with the practice of fasting. Throughout history, the salu-
brious health benefits of fasting appeared in a strangely
diverse array of history books, literature, and medical
textbooks. The Greek physician Hippocrates made refer-
ence to the healing properties of fasting, "Everyone has a
doctor in him; we just have to help him in his work. The
natural healing force within each one of us is the greatest force in getting well . . . to eat when you are sick, is to
feed your sickness." Other famous people have touted the
health-promoting properties of fasting throughout history, including Ben Franklin, who was rumored to have
said, "The best of all medicines is resting and fasting."
Mark Twain wrote, "A little starvation can really do more

for the average sick man than can the best medicines and the best doctors."

Historically, the therapeutic value of fasting is tied to epilepsy more than to any other disease. Epilepsy had confused, fascinated and frustrated physicians as far back as the Egyptians. Epilepsy comes from ancient Greek, meaning "to seize, possess, or afflict." The Greeks also called epilepsy the "sacred disease" and as civilizations before them, they viewed it as a form of spiritual possession. The eccentric, clumsy and bizarre treatments that followed were a reflection of epilepsy's mysterious and unknown origin. "Surely patients with no other disease have grasped at so many therapeutic straws," wrote one physician in the 1920's. Doctors' attempts to quell epileptic fits were a patchwork of trial and error: bloodletting, trephining of the skull (boring a hole in the skull to release the disease), removal of the ovaries and adrenal glands, countless drugs, herbs, and tinctures. When the Roman physician Celsus witnessed epileptics drinking blood from the wounds of dying gladiators he wrote, "What a miserable disease that makes tolerable such a miserable remedy." By the 1920s drinking blood was no longer suggested as cure but little else had changed. "Many Modern 'cures' are not less miserable" wrote a respected neurologist, comparing the state of treatment in the 1920s to those of the past.

Leading up to the 1920s, the "modern" therapies for epilepsy consisted of two drugs: bromine and Luminal (phenobarbital). Both drugs were only marginally good at preventing seizures, and came with a mosaic of side effects coupled with heavy sedation. Then, in 1920, Hugh Conklin, a drugless osteopathic physician working out of Battle Creek Sanitarium in Battle Creek Michigan, claimed he had found a cure for epilepsy.

In the late teens and 20s, sanitariums were an *en vogue* destination for people suffering from any ailment, perceived or otherwise. The masses boarded trains to Battle Creek to visit sanitariums where they would receive enemas, soak in mineral water baths, sunbathe nude, and *fast*. Conklin boldly claimed a "water only" fast of 20 days was a sure-fire cure for epilepsy. Conklin's claim eventually rippled outward to more conventional physicians on the east coast, prompting Rawle Geyelin, a highly respected endocrinologist at New York Presbyterian Hospital, to test Conklin's claim. In 1921, Geyelin presented his findings to a packed audience at the annual American Medical Association convention: after fasting 30 patients for 20 days in his clinic: 87 percent of the patients became seizure free.

One of the patients Geyelin treated was the son of a wealthy New York attorney named Charles Howland. His son had failed conventional treatment with drugs, and paid a heavy price in side effects. After Geyelin's fasting treatment cured his son with none of the side effects of drugs, Howland was shocked and inspired enough to write a check for five thousand dollars (a lot of money for the time) to John Hopkins to study why fasting worked. At Hopkins, researchers collected and exhaustively analyzed urine and blood samples taken from fasting patients detailed every observation—from water loss, to electrolyte balance, to acid/base balance, and curiously, the mention of the occurrence of two small ketone molecules, *beta-hydroxybutyrate and acetoacetate,* in the fasting patient's plasma and urine. To the researchers at Hopkins, the compounds were a mystery. In the end they concluded they were a meaningless waste product; the byproduct of the "incomplete oxidation of fats."

In the summer of 1921, at the Mayo Clinic in Rochester Minnesota, a doctor named Russell Wilder published three short paragraphs in The Clinical Bulletin. "It has occurred to us that the benefit of Dr. Geyelin's procedure may be dependent on the *ketonemia* [high blood levels of ketones in the blood] which must result from such fasts, and that possibly equally good results could be obtained if a ketonemia were produced by some other means," wrote Wilder. Wilder was speculating that ketones (beta-hydroxybutyrate and acetoacetate) generated from fasting might be more than merely metabolic waste, that they might be of unrecognized significance. Perhaps it was ketones themselves, reasoned Wilder, that were behind the levees protecting against the electrical tidal waves inside the brains of fasting epileptics. Others had shown that the ketones generated by fasting could also be achieved by a low carbohydrate and high fat diet—*the nutritional maintenance of the fasting state.* Wilder was anxious to test his theory. "It is proposed, therefore, to try the effect of such *ketogenic diets* on a series of epileptics."

Mynie Peterman, a Mayo Clinic pediatrician, decided to test Wilder's hypothesis by setting up a clinical trial. He decided to select children as participants given their generally poor response to the only two drugs available at the time coupled with their higher risk of dire side effects. Peterman followed 37 children on the ketogenic diet for periods of time ranging from 4 months up to two-and-a-half years. All tallied, 60 percent of the children became seizure free, 34.5 percent were improved, and 5.5 percent showed no response. The ketogenic diet was a resounding success—undeniably better than the existing drugs. The news swept across the country and the diet and became the new standard of care for pediatric epilepsy. As more and more physicians began adopting it as a treatment, the contrast between the ketogenic diet and the heavily-sedative, anti-seizure drugs was easily observed. "The diet is well tolerated without causing any untoward symptoms in the patients. On the contrary, they seem to be more alert and less nervous," commented one physician.

Yet the diet's tenure was short-lived. By the late 1930s, pharmaceutical chemists isolated anti-seizure drugs with somewhat more tolerable side effects than previous anti-seizure medications. Parke-Davis presented the results of its new drug Dilantin claiming it was able to eliminate, or greatly reduce the seizures in 74 percent of the children and adults treated. Minor toxic symptoms were reported in 15 percent of the patients and "more serious toxic reactions" were reported in 5 percent. Dilantin became available in the summer of 1938.

Not surprisingly, physicians found Dilatin much easier to implement (and more lucrative) than the ketogenic diet. The popularity of the drug grew quickly. By 1940 it was hailed as ushering in a new epoch in the treatment of epilepsy. One doctor called it "the most remarkable and important chemotherapeutic agent in the convulsive disorders since 1912." The success of Dilantin inspired other pharmaceutical companies to quickly establish their own in-house, large-scale drug screening programs. The massively scaled-up efforts produced results. Over the next two decades, a dozen new anticonvulsants hit the pharmacy shelves.

The rest is history. With a flood of easy-to-pop pills, the ketogenic diet vanished from the clinic and then from the literature. No trials were ever performed to determine if the ketogenic diet was a better front-line treatment than the anti-seizure drugs (even though the majority of data suggests that it is). Physicians today still comment on the remarkable difference between children placed on a ketogenic diet and those on anti-seizure drugs. The children on the ketogenic diet appear much sharper and less sedated, and many of them reach developmental milestones that once seemed out of their grasp. The diet was shown to marginally affect linear growth but many catch up on some or all of the lost ground. Yet none of this seemed to matter: The drugs were simply too convenient. By the time Cahill became interested in ketones in the 1960s, the ketogenic diet as a treatment for pediatric epilepsy was nothing more than a footnote in a few medical textbooks.

In fact, as Cahill noted, for the majority of the twentieth century, ketone metabolism was almost exclusively associated not with epilepsy but instead with a pathological condition known as *ketoacidosis*. Ketoacidosis occurs most frequently in people with type 1 diabetes (and poorly controlled type 2 diabetes) who are unable to produce their own insulin. With insulin at dangerously low levels, the liver is unable to regulate blood glucose levels leading to high levels of circulating glucose and subsequent aberrant ketone production. The flood of ketones results in an acidification of the blood. If not treated quickly, ketoacidosis can result in coma and death. The ketogenic diet became guilty by association.

Researchers knew by the mid-1920s that ketone bodies were a metabolic fuel—the fourth fuel—but for inexplicable reasons medical textbooks always framed ketones in the context of a pathological state—either as a dangerous consequence of starving, or worse, as life-threatening ketoacidosis. As the century wore on, little changed. By mid-century, the "fat is bad" dietary mantra had taken hold and the ketogenic diet, high in fat, was seen as a terribly unhealthy diet. Most physicians and researchers viewed the presence of ketone bodies in the blood was a result of "faulty metabolism."

An undergraduate biochemistry textbook from 1995 succinctly described the prevailing sentiment of ketone metabolism (Albert Lehninger, the co-discoverer of mitochondria as the site of oxidative phosphorylation, was one of three authors). "In individuals on very low-calorie diets, fats stored in adipose tissue become the major energy source. The levels of ketone bodies in the blood and urine should be monitored to avoid the dangers of acidosis and ketosis." In 1995, ketosis, even in a healthy person under a low-calorie or fasted state, was considered dangerous—a pathological state of metabolism that was best avoided.

Reading through the publications on ketosis over the twentieth century, it is clear that Cahill was one of the first to look at ketosis through a different lens. As is often the case in science, the first step to progress is simply the act of questioning dogmatic assumptions. Cahill began to question the pervasive assumption that ketosis was nothing more than a perversion of normal metabolism that appeared when someone was sick with diabetes or dying from starvation. Critically, Cahill began to view ketosis as an elegant evolutionary adaptation to the inevitable periods when our ancestors didn't have access to food— an auxiliary engine using a fuel that kicked in when we needed it the most. This change in perception compelled him to ask more questions. If indeed ketosis was an adaptation to starvation, might ketone metabolism be a *normal*, perfectly safe form of metabolism? Perhaps, ketones even evolved into a *more efficient* fuel to limp us through hard times?

Luckily for Cahill, he was asking these questions in the late 1950s and 60s when therapeutic fasting was a common treatment for obesity and Institutional Review Board (IRB) committees were much more permissive about human experimentation. It was fairly routine for doctors to therapeutically fast (water-only fast) patients with obesity desperate to lose weight, sometimes for months on end (The longest fast on record occurred in 1965 when a 27-year-old Scotsman with obesity went 382 days with nothing but water, tea and black coffee).

Cahill knew that the fasting metabolism in humans came with a theoretical problem: the brain. Our brains, relative to other species, are massive metabolic sinks, consuming up to 20 percent of the body's available energy while at rest. In children, it's even higher; up to 50 percent of available energy is consumed by the brain. In Cahill's time, it was thought the brain was metabolically inflexible. It was assumed that the brain relied solely on glucose as a fuel. Researchers knew that most of the body's tissues could oxidize fats for fuel but the blood-brain barrier blocked most large molecules—like fatty acids—from crossing into the brain. The problem, then, for a fasting human came down to one of storage. A person only stored about a one-day supply of glucose in the form of glycogen in the liver and muscle. (Muscle glycogen stores much more glucose than the liver but it is only accessible to muscle tissue.) Once a person stops eating and burns through their stored supply, then what? During a fast, how did the body maintain a constant level of blood glucose to feed the voracious appetite of the brain? Biochemists knew that certain amino acids could be cannibalized from muscle and converted into glucose (a process called gluconeogenesis) but this obviously could not go on for long because the person would progressively lose more and more muscle until they wasted away and died. When Cahill did the math, the extent of the problem was revealed: a fasting person under "normal" metabolic conditions would be expected to die in about 18 days. Yet clearly that was not the case. A normal weight person could fast for about two months, and as the Scotsman just demonstrated, an obese person could go over a year without even a single bite of food.

To answer these questions, Cahill performed a series of experiments on otherwise healthy people with obesity after they had fasted for 40 days. To learn more about ketosis, Cahill needed to get a snapshot of the entirety of ketone metabolism within the body. Specifically, he needed to concurrently measure the different metabolites organs were producing and consuming after adapting to a starvation state. To do this, he and Oliver Owen, a medical resident, simultaneously inserted catheters into the blood vessels entering and exiting the subject's kidneys, liver and brain. This procedure was not without risk. "Although our team at the cardiac catheterization laboratory had provided for every safety precaution, we were concerned about the inherent risks of obtaining multiple artery and venous blood samples from a patient who had not eaten for 41 days," wrote Owen. In the end, they performed the experiment of three subjects without incident.

According to Cahill's results, the conversion to ketosis goes like this: once a person stops eating, the body turns to its stores of liver glycogen. This lasts for about twenty-four hours. Once depleted of this stored carbohydrate, the body now faces a crisis. There are certain cells in the body (red blood cells, corneal cells and small neurons in the brain) that have no mitochondria and therefore have only one metabolic pathway available to supply energy: glycolysis. Glycolysis requires glucose. So, with no glucose coming in through diet, and all the stores of glucose spent, the body has to come up with a way to maintain a base level of blood glucose, about 80 grams per day, to feed these glucose-dependent cells. Cahill's experiments showed that the body does this by patching together several contributory pathways. The liver and kidneys orchestrate the process, cobbling together glucose production by pulling metabolites from other pathways and converting them into glucose, with some glucose made from pyruvate and lactate, some made from glycerol (a 3-carbon molecule that is cleaved off of triglycerides prior to the oxidation of fats), some from certain amino acids, some from the Krebs cycle intermediate oxaloacetate and some from ketones themselves.

Even with the multitude of pathways providing glucose, there was still the problem of the brain. Cahill knew from simple calculations that if brain function was indeed totally reliant on glucose, it would quickly drain the supply being generated from the patchwork of pathways. To measure the fuels entering and leaving the brain, Cahill inserted catheters into the fasting subjects' carotid arteries and jugular veins. What he discovered solved the metabolic dilemma presented by the fasting brain: "As we expected, [it] showed some two thirds of brain fuel consumption to be D-β-hydroxybutyrate and acetoacetate." This changed the math. By showing that the brain could pivot from glucose to ketones for fuel, the metabolic dilemma posed by the fasting human was solved. Nobel Laureate Harold Varmus once said, "I soon learned how much more important a new measurement was than an old theory." Indeed, this new measurement, showing the brain was not exclusively reliant on glucose and could transition to burning ketone bodies—changed everything.

Cahill's research illuminated the entire metabolic conversion to ketosis that is set in motion when a person stops eating. Insulin provides the key signal. With no carbohydrate stimulating the release of insulin, fat cells are quickly mobilized, releasing triglycerides into the bloodstream. This solves the food shortage for the many tissues that are able to use fatty acids for energy through a process called beta-oxidation that takes place in the mitochondria. A fatty acid is a chain of linked carbon atoms with varying numbers of hydrogen atoms attached along the chain (Fats with more hydrogens are called saturated fats and those with fewer hydrogens are unsaturated fats). The *beta* in beta-oxidation refers to the second carbon atom in from the end of the chain. For beta-oxidation to occur, enzymes first cut the fatty acid chain at the beta carbon bond, producing a two-carbon molecule called *acetate* that combines with coenzyme A to form acetyl-coA. Acetyl-coA can then enter the Krebs cycle → electron transport chain → ATP.

The hepatocytes in the liver act as the manufacturing line for ketone bodies. They do the work of pumping out ketone bodies primarily to meet the voracious energy appetite of the brain. Fatty acids enter hepatocytes and start the process of beta-oxidation, generating acetyl-CoA. But here's the critical difference between normal carbohydrate metabolism and what happens as a result of the shift to ketosis in liver cells: during ketosis, the final product of the Krebs cycle, oxaloacetate, is pulled from the cycle and shuttled through a gluconeogenic pathway to help generate glucose. With little oxaloacetate to bind with acetyl-coA (the final step in the Krebs cycle), the pool of acetyl-coA begins to build up. The enzyme that converts acetyl-coA into the ketone body acetoacetate is freely floating around in the mitochondrial matrix, just waiting to do its job. Now, with acetyl-coA *spilling over* into the mitochondrial matrix, this enzyme begins converting the excess acetyl-coA into acetoacetate. Another enzyme then converts acetoacetate into beta-hydroxybutyrate. Finally, beta-hydroxybutyrate and acetoacetate are released into the circulation as water-soluble molecules (about 2/3 BHB, 1/3 acetoacetate and a negligible amount of acetone generated from acetoacetate spontaneously breaking down).

The brain isn't the only organ that then imports and burns the ketone bodies circulating in the blood—the heart and muscle do, too. The metabolic transition to ketosis, Cahill then showed, has a built-in mechanism that regulates the entire process—an elegant feedback loop of regulatory control. The accumulation of beta-hydroxybutyrate in the blood circles back to adipose tissue and signals for it to slow down the release of triglycerides into the bloodstream, thus ensuring fuel is efficiently metered out only as needed.

What Cahill revealed was a finely tuned auxiliary metabolism that is hidden inside of all of us. Far from pathological, it has been *essential* to our survival. "Thus, a normal adult human could survive two months of starvation; an obese person could survive much longer," wrote Cahill. "Were it not for the β-hydroxybutyrate and acetoacetate providing brain fuel, we Homo sapiens might not be here!"

In truth, what Cahill had revealed was two distinct forms of metabolism—one that operated under a standard American diet, heavy in carbohydrate intake, and the other that operated under conditions of fasting, extreme calorie restriction, or a very-low-carbohydrate ketogenic diet. The difference centered on the activity of the hormone insulin and the liver. "Thus we can think of the liver as working in one of two modes: a low-insulin state characterized by gluconeogenesis, lipolysis [fat burning], and ketogenesis; and a high-insulin state characterized by glycolysis, lipogenesis [fat synthesizing], and fat export. In the former, the liver's energy is provided by beta-oxidation of fatty acids; in the latter state, the tricarboxylic acid cycle produces the energy."

The looming question now was this: Does ketosis have benefits outside of mere survival? It was already discovered (and forgotten) that fasting and/or a ketogenic diet was an extraordinarily effective treatment for epilepsy. *Were there other conditions that might benefit from the shift to ketone metabolism?*

Cahill's reimaging of ketosis as a non-pathological and perfectly normal metabolic state faced an uphill battle. During the 80s and 90s the "fat is bad" mantra was hitting full stride. Therapeutic fasting was replaced by bariatric surgery. The FDA urged people to avoid fat, especially saturated fats. The aisles of grocery stores quickly filled with low-fat alternatives to real food. Cahill's message was lost in the noise. The idea of fasting and a high-fat ketogenic diet was vehemently rejected by the vast majority of dieticians and physicians across the country. "Ketones," was still a dirty word. This was the state of the science of ketosis when Veech's laboratory banked everything on the expectation that studying ketosis would reveal something truly important, something deemed useful to the NIH reviewers.

Veech set out to answer the questions that Cahill's research had inspired: Does ketosis have additional benefits beyond its role as an auxiliary fuel? Veech and his colleagues decided the best way to answer this question was to compare ketone metabolism to the "normal" physiological conditions associated with a standard American diet. Specifically, he would measure cellular metabolic parameters of heart muscle fed under three separate conditions: glucose alone, glucose plus insulin and glucose plus ketones. These conditions, reasoned Veech, should be a good way to compare the "typical" cellular metabolism that occurs when people eat a normal, high carbohydrate diet to metabolism while in the state of ketosis. Under "normal" circumstances, after each meal, blood glucose spikes are followed by the release of insulin from the pancreas. The primary job of insulin is to lower blood sugar by signaling the cell to "open up." Insulin signals a transport protein called GLUT4 to embed itself into the cellular membrane and allow glucose to diffuse into the cell.

Additionally, insulin signals for the cell to speed up the conversion of pyruvate to acetyl-coA. The conversion of pyruvate to acetyl-coA is done by a large multi enzyme complex called the pyruvate dehydrogenase complex (PDH). PDH is a metabolic gatekeeper. It responds to cellular signals like insulin by controlling the rate that pyruvate enters the Krebs cycle. The important point is this: under a typical high-carbohydrate American diet, insulin is controlling the flux of metabolites that enter the Krebs cycle. This flux determines how "charged" the controlling nucleotide coenzymes are that drive our metabolism: ATP, NAD+, NADP+, and Acetyl-coA. When eating a standard American diet, these spikes in glucose followed by the release of insulin are repeated throughout the day with each meal and snack.

On the other hand, ketone metabolism achieved through fasting or a ketogenic diet is devoid of the spikes in blood sugar and the concomitant insulin release. It is characterized by a typically lower and steadier blood glucose level as the metabolism patches together sources of glucose to maintain the necessary baseline level of blood glucose. Therefore, to match real metabolic conditions of the body in the state of ketosis, Veech just added ketones and a steady concentration of glucose without insulin.

What they discovered was paradigm shifting. When the heart tissue was given glucose with no insulin, the muscular work performed per unit of oxygen consumed—a direct measure of energy efficiency in heart muscle—was just 10 percent. Next, when a saturating dose of insulin was added to the glucose, the metabolic efficiency of the heart muscle jumped to 28 percent. Last, when they tested ketone bodies and glucose together (mimicking natural conditions under ketosis), the efficiency essentially matched that of glucose plus a saturating dose of insulin at 25 percent. The take home message was this: ketone bodies are a *remarkably* potent fuel—increasing metabolic efficiency from 10 percent with glucose alone, to 25 percent when BHB is added. This *single distinction* is the fulcrum that all of the magical properties of BHB pivot upon.

The reason ketones are so metabolically efficient is the fact they are a thermodynamically superior fuel. Every fuel is uniquely imbued with a different amount of potential energy within its bonds. For example, a car can travel further when burning one gallon of regular gasoline compared to one gallon of ethanol-containing gasoline, because ethanol contains less energy per unit volume. Ketones hold the same advantage. Ketones have more starting energy per two-carbon unit than glucose. This is measured by something called the heat of combustion that tallies the total amount of energy in any given fuel. D-β-hydroxybutyrate contains −1021 kJ/mole whereas glucose contains only −933 kJ/mole (the more negative the number, the more energy). Critically, Veech's research showed that the increased energy stored within BHB was captured by the electron transport chain and translated into a more *charged* ATP.

Recall the electron transport chain. Remember that NADH feeds electrons into complex I. The electrons then travel to the Coenzyme Q couple and the energy from the transfer is captured by ejecting a proton into the intermembrane space of the mitochondria, creating Mitchell's chemiosmotic gradient that, in turn, generates ATP. Under ketosis, the ratio of mitochondrial NADH to NAD is increased; in other words, the NADH/NAD battery is more charged. And second, the Coenzyme Q couple is more oxidized. In effect, this "widens the energetic gap" between complex I and the Coenzyme Q couple, with the result of ejecting the proton into the intermembrane space with more force. This results in a *stronger* chemiosmotic gradient and *more* ATP production. It is as if the distance between complex I and the Coenzyme Q couple is a waterfall and the machinery ejecting the proton into the intermembrane space is the waterwheel. Ketosis *heightens* the waterfall, providing more energy to the waterwheel. In effect, ketones were able to "supercharge" the cell, said Veech.

The details of Veech's study raised another question. BHB was much more efficient than glucose alone, but essentially *equally* efficient when a saturating dose of insulin was added. At first glance, one might be forgiven for not being overly impressed—ketones are as efficient as glucose plus a saturating dose of insulin—25 percent versus 28 percent, respectively. A saturating dose of insulin, however, does not reflect *normal* physiological conditions. Looking closer—as Cahill and Veech reflected on the results in a broader context—they began to realize that the shift to ketone metabolism for the majority of the adult population held a profound therapeutic potential. Here is why: a standard American diet, compared to the state of ketosis, resulted in two very different metabolic outcomes. First, consider the standard American diet: in between high-carbohydrate meals, when insulin is lower and the metabolism is idling along at its basal metabolic rate, metabolic efficiency (output per unit oxygen) is a paltry 10 percent. This means all of the nucleotide coenzymes are less charged and the entirety of metabolism operates less efficiently. Second, over time, almost everyone eating a high-carbohydrate diet combined with a low-level of activity will develop something called insulin resistance (highly-active people eating a high-carb diet are much less susceptible to developing insulin resistance—active muscle will freely "soak up" blood glucose thus reducing the need of insulin). Insulin resistance, however, is more the norm than the exception in America—over half of the adults have some measurable degree of insulin resistance.

Insulin resistance is just as it sounds: the cell becomes resistant to the effects of insulin and is progressively less efficient at shuttling glucose from the bloodstream into the cell and is less able to metabolize glucose efficiently as the pyruvate dehydrogenase complex also becomes less responsive to insulin. The consequence of this pernicious process is that the metabolic efficiency Veech measured with glucose and a saturating dose of insulin at 28 percent, begins to drop. The upshot: all four nucleotide coenzymes are less *charged* and less able to efficiently drive metabolism. The thousands of reactions that comprised human metabolism sputter and slow.

The magic of ketosis, Veech and Cahill realized, is that it *always* achieves a metabolic efficiency of 25 percent. In other words, ketone metabolism effectively "supercharges" our basal metabolism, taking the efficiency from 10 percent to 25 percent. Second, and this is critically important, ketone metabolism bypasses a myriad of problems associated with insulin resistance. There is no such thing as "ketone resistance." Ketones enter the cell through an entirely different transport protein than the insulin-controlled glucose transport protein, GLUT4. And they also bypass the insulin-controlled pyruvate dehydrogenase complex by entering metabolism further downstream. Herein lies the magic of ketosis: by entering the cell through a different route—and by-passing the pyruvate dehydrogenase complex—ketone metabolism is able to *completely side-step* the insulin dependent pathways—analogous to an open lane on a traffic-jammed freeway.

In strict metabolic terms, as we age, due to insulin resistance, our metabolism becomes less and less efficient. Under ketosis, however, the metabolic efficiency can be sustained at a remarkably high 25 percent. The effect of ketosis, then, is that the four "great" controlling nucleotide coenzymes—the central hubs of metabolic activity that power the entire metabolic map—are much more charged. The results of this study arced back to his work in Krebs laboratory—the realization that beta-hydroxybutyrate could change the ratios of the four "controlling" nucleotide coenzymes wove his career into a single, harmonious continuum. In terms of metabolism, this new fuel affects *everything*. For example, the synthesis of serotonin, the "feel-good," social neurotransmitter, is powered by NADPH. Under ketosis, NADPH is more charged and thus able to drive the reactions of serotonin synthesis further. The result: more serotonin. Your mood lightens; you have a greater sense of well-being and exhibit less compulsive behavior. Dopamine, another neurotransmitter responsible for a sense of well-being, is also geared to NADPH. Operating through the four nucleotide coenzymes over a thousand metabolic reactions are pushed to further completion under ketosis. The chemical motion that pushes back against entropy; the chemical motion that *defines* life, is amplified by this single, simple fuel. The therapeutic potential, realized Veech, was enormous. "Understanding the control of metabolic pathways by the "great" controlling nucleotide coenzyme couples and changes in their chemical energies by the simple metabolite d-β-hydroxybutyrate offer new biochemical and therapeutic opportunities. These opportunities include increasing the efficiency of aerobic exercise, treating diseases of insulin resistance, combating reactive oxygen toxicity and extending lifespan," wrote Veech.

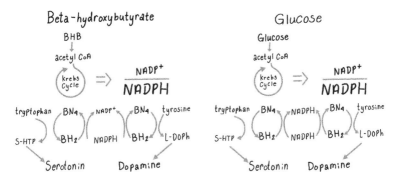

Figure illustrating how burning BHB compared to glucose increases the ratio of NADPH to NADP+ (*charging* it more) and therefore drives the metabolic reactions "coupled" or "geared" to NADPH further, generating more neurotransmitters like serotonin and dopamine.

Veech's illumination of this previously maligned and hidden form of metabolism had curiously far-reaching clinical potential. Ketosis, Veech realized, offered a solution to our sorry metabolic state. Maybe ketosis should be our default condition if we want to side-step insulin resistance, diabetes, dementia, Alzheimer's and other chronic diseases. Perhaps ketosis, however achieved, promises a new, more graceful way to age. As Veech reflected, he began to realize that the therapeutic implications appeared almost too good to be true. "What are the potential uses of BHB in addition to pediatric epilepsy? Theoretically, any condition wherein oxygen supply to cells may be limited. This list would encompass almost *every disease state*," wrote Veech and Cahill.

For Veech's laboratory, however, the remarkable findings on ketone metabolism turned out to be too little too late in the eyes of the NIH reviewers. The writing was already on the wall, "They had already moved him into an office that looked like a broom closet," said an associate. At the end of the two years, they made the decision to stop funding his work. "By the time the work defining the metabolic effects of ketones and insulin on glycolytic and mitochondrial metabolism was published, my laboratory had been closed, and its workers and techniques had been dispersed. As an overage civil servant, I could not be 'fired' but had no other visible means of support," wrote Veech. Veech used this time to take a sabbatical and "reflect on the implications of our findings on the remarkable effects of ketone bodies." He knew he faced an uphill battle. With his NIH funding gone, it wasn't clear if the therapeutic aspect of ketosis would be realized anytime soon. "Krebs once remarked that it usually takes about a generation for advances in basic science to be applied in medicine. This has certainly been the case in applying our understanding of the linked network of equilibria involving the great nucleotide systems," lamented Veech.

By the turn of the century, the climate surrounding dietary recommendation and nutrition science was showing stirrings of change. Dr. Atkins released his book *Diet Revolution* in 1972, making the heretical suggestion that it was the carbohydrates—bread, pasta, rice and sugar—that was responsible for America's expanding waistline. He boldly suggested that fat was a "neutral" food. The timing was terrible, however. Dr. Atkins was ridiculed, slandered and labeled a quack. Nevertheless, his message proved surprisingly resilient. Especially among the many people who had experienced firsthand the potent weight-loss effect of Atkins diet. Eventually, a few mavericks began outright questioning the foundation of the government's food pyramid. In 2002, the New York Times published an article by science journalist (and self-proclaimed "nutrition heretic"), Gary Taubes, titled *What if It's All Been a Big Fat Lie?* The investigative piece was a scathing review of the existing dietary recommendations that pushed carbohydrates and vilified fat. He systematically questioned the dietary advice of the American Medical Association and the American Heart Association and presented convincing evidence that this misguided advice might be underpinning America's obesity and type 2 diabetes epidemic.

According to Taubes, the dietary recommendations were upside down and backward. Remember, the switch to tell the body to burn fat and manufacture ketones is low insulin, but the high carbohydrate intake suggested by the dietary recommendations resulted in large spikes in insulin throughout the day. Once in the cell, glucose can either enter the glycolytic pathway to be used for fuel or, if present in excess, it will enter the lipogenic pathway and be converted to fat for storage. So, said Taubes, with the standard American diet we are essentially shutting down fat burning and turning up fat generation. "As a result [of eating high-glycemic foods], they cause a spike of blood sugar and a surge of insulin within minutes. The resulting rush of insulin stores the blood sugar away and a few hours later, your blood sugar is lower than it was before you ate . . . your body effectively thinks it has run out of fuel, but the insulin is still high enough to prevent you from burning your own fat. The result is hunger and a craving for more carbohydrates. It's another vicious circle, and another situation ripe for obesity," wrote Taubes.

The Atkins diet is essentially a ketogenic diet. Dr. Atkins, Taubes explained, was an early adopter of Cahill's suggestion that ketosis might be a good thing. Atkins liked to "say that ketosis was so energizing that it was better than sex, which set him up for some ridicule. An inevitable criticism of Atkins's diet has been that ketosis is dangerous and to be avoided at all costs," wrote Taubes.

Taubes then cited an interview with Veech: "When I interviewed ketosis experts, however, they universally sided with Atkins, and suggested that maybe the medical community and the media confuse ketosis with ketoacidosis, a variant of ketosis that occurs in untreated diabetics and can be fatal. 'Doctors are scared of ketosis,' says Richard Veech, an N.I.H. researcher who studied medicine at Harvard and then got his doctorate at Oxford University with the Nobel Laureate Hans Krebs. 'They're always worried about diabetic ketoacidosis. But ketosis is a normal physiologic state. I would argue it is the normal state of man. It's not normal to have McDonald's and a delicatessen around every corner. It's normal to starve.'"

Veech's suggestion that ketosis might be "the normal state of man," in the New York Times was a big stride forward. Yet, the inertia established by the government food pyramid, the food industry, and all the physicians and scientists who held the party line, would not be turned around by a single article. But the tide was shifting. Veech, however, was still without funding. That was about to change.

In the early 2000s, Dr. Joseph Bielitzki, the Veterinarian Chief at NASA received a call from the Defense Advanced Research Project Agency (DARPA). He had acquired a reputation for creative ideas while at NASA. Word of his reputation made its way to the higher-ups at DARPA and they offered him a job as a program manager. "Most of the Program Managers are brought in by invitation for a two to four-year period. Some of them may stay six, but pretty much you're brought in for new ideas and then you're let go because you've run out of them," said Bielitzki. DARPA was not interested in small ideas. Their mission was to gain a military advantage and this required bold thinking. "Well, DARPA's a little bit different because they don't tell you what you have to work on. Your job is to also determine what you want to work on. It has to have military relevance, it has to be forward-thinking, you can't be incremental, it has to be more revolutionary than evolutionary," said Bielitzki.

When Bielitzki arrived in Washington, DC, shortly after the 9/11 terror attacks, the US military was involved in Iraq and Afghanistan. One of the problems confronting the military was physical endurance. "One of the issues was how do you provide support to the war fighter, the young men and women who were going out into the field of combat in these places that really are pretty hostile environments when you think about working in 120 degrees, carrying 90 pounds, you don't wear body armor, and all the protective clothing and equipment you've gotta carry, so one of the questions was, if we're gonna put them in that condition, how do we make sure that they have adequate calories that they can do their task, not become fatigued and not set them up to fail at a time when it's critical to their life?"

The timing was fortuitous. Bielitzki was an amateur triathlete and had a growing interest in ways to increase the efficiency of aerobic energy metabolism. "It's swim/

cycle/run and the fourth sport of triathlons is nutrition," said Bielitzki. "How do you fuel yourself over that five hours you're doing that half Ironman or that 10 hours you're doing that full Ironman? Nutrition is an art and a science in and of itself." This led Bielitzki to Veech's paper showing ketone metabolism can increase the efficiency of muscle by 25 percent. Although it was still early, and decidedly against the prevailing wisdom that endurance sports required ample carbohydrates, Bielitzki was intrigued—it was exactly the kind of out-of-the-box idea that DARPA was known for. "Everybody that works with DARPA thinks the Program Managers are crazy, to some extent. You're expected to be off-the-wall, you're expected to push the envelope beyond where it could be and people say it's out-of-the-box thinking and I used to tell them, 'We don't even believe there is a box.' So, how far can you push it? We knew butyric was an end product of fat metabolism; that's where it enters the Krebs cycle, so it was a rational, logical place to look," said Bielitzki.

Bielitzki contacted Veech and a biochemist named Kieran Clarke at Oxford. "Both of them have pedigrees in metabolic physiology that you're not gonna replicate very many places," said Bielitzki. The three of them proposed a project to DARPA. The grant was awarded. Ten million dollars. The irony was not lost on Veech. The NIH, which had cut off his funding, was the institute with the mission to improve health and cure disease. And a defense agency, with an entirely different mission, had stepped in to fund Veech's work. "NIH have never given money for this kind of metabolic research. DARPA wanted it because they wanted to improve the performance of the special forces," said Veech.

The grant was to develop a ketone ester that would induce ketosis upon ingestion. It would then be tested for safety and its ability to improve endurance for warfighters. But it didn't stop there. The money was also dedicated for more altruistic purposes. The award abstract stated: "In addition to the military uses of such compounds, it appears that mild ketosis would be of therapeutic benefit in 3 major disease phenotypes: 1) diseases of substrate deficiency, such as Alzheimer's disease, types I & II diabetes, and insulin resistant states, 2) diseases of free radical toxicity, such as Parkinson's disease, amyotrophic lateral sclerosis and reperfusion injury and 3) diseases of hypoxia, such as myocardial infarction and stroke."

Veech was not alone in his belief in the therapeutic possibilities surrounding ketosis. Cahill, too, who spent his entire career studying the corrosive effects of insulin resistance and type 2 diabetes, understood the profound therapeutic potential inherent to ketosis. Cahill was intimately aware that the corrosive cascade—starting with insulin resistance leading to prediabetes and finally clinically overt type 2 diabetes—exacted an enormous toll on the health of the global population and taxed the health care system to the tune of billions of dollars every year. Worse, Alzheimer's disease was beginning to be understood as yet another manifestation of this same process. A PET scan, which measures glucose uptake in the brain, clearly shows the Alzheimer's patient's brain is unable to efficiently utilize glucose. In effect, the brain is *starving*. Studies have shown that those with type 2 diabetes have double the risk of developing Alzheimer's. For that reason, some clinicians have now begun to refer to Alzheimer's as "type 3 diabetes," acknowledging the contribution of insulin resistance to this devastating disease. Ketosis—Veech and Cahill realized—could theoretically solve both of these pernicious problems by simply bypassing the entire pathology inherent to the brain of an Alzheimer's victim. Or better yet, preventing it from happening in the first place.

In 2001 Cahill and Veech coauthored a paper titled "Ketone Bodies, Potential Therapeutic Uses." The paper ran through the underlying logic suggesting that the metabolic state of ketosis had the potential to mitigate a remarkable range of disease processes. Indeed, the potential to treat Alzheimer's was particularly seductive: "Given the body of evidence already existing showing the therapeutic efficacy of ketone bodies in a variety of conditions, a direct study involving ketone therapy seems warranted."

Veech and Cahill suggested that the best route to testing ketone bodies on diseases like Alzheimer's was to develop a food-like product that could readily raise blood ketone levels. "Clinical maneuvers for increasing blood levels of Beta-hydroxybutyrate to 2–5 mmol may require synthetic esters or polymers of BHB taken orally, probably 100 to 150 g or more daily. This necessitates advances in food-science technology." The "ketone-ester," suggested by Veech and Cahill, is a clever way to get BHB into the body. As it turns out, simply manufacturing BHB is not an easy task. The first problem in manufacturing *exogenous* ketones, as they are often referred to, is that BHB is an acid. For an acid to be made edible it is usually conjugated as a salt, meaning the BHB is attached to a positive ion like sodium, calcium, potassium or magnesium. Unfortunately, to achieve the blood levels Veech thought to be therapeutic, would require ingesting very high levels of these salts, far beyond recommended amounts. Additionally, ketone salt supplements typically come as a mixture of two different enantiomeric forms of BHB, the L-form and the D-form. An enantiomer is a mirror image of the same molecule. For example, your left and your right hand are enantiomers—mirror images of each other. When fasting or adhering to a ketogenic diet, the body produces the D-form of BHB exclusively. The L-form ends up being burned like a fat through the beta oxidation pathway, entering the electron transport chain through complex II. Only the D-form is able to widen the energetic gap by entering the electron transport chain through complex I and increasing the energetic span between complex I and the coenzyme Q couple—resulting in a reduction of free radical production and the hyper-charging the four critical coenzyme couples. Veech realized that a ketone ester solved both of the problems inherent to manufacturing ketone supplements. It circumvents the need to conjugate BHB as a salt and contains only the D-form of BHB. The ester, with the technical name D-beta-hydroxybutyrate-(R)-1,3 butanediol monoester, consists of one molecule of D-BHB attached to a D-BHB precursor molecule that is cleaved off and converted to D-BHB in the liver, thus releasing two molecules of D-BHB.

"IT FELT LIKE A LIGHT SWITCH HAD COME ON"

F
inally, flush with money, Veech could get back to his lab. In order to realize the dream of the ester, there was a lot of work to do. In their 2001 paper, Cahill and Veech acknowledged that because no viable therapy for Alzheimer's currently existed, patients faced a grim scenario. But the metabolic conversion to ketosis, according to their research, exhibited much promise as a treatment for Alzheimer's. The science of ketosis, "Gave hope that new therapies may soon be available for this currently untreatable disease," they wrote. With those who were presently facing this grim prognosis there was no time to wait for the ester to be developed. This was the position a medical doctor named Mary Newport found herself in when her husband was diagnosed with Alzheimer's disease in 2005.

In 2001 it became obvious to Mary Newport, a practicing neonatologist, that something was off about her husband Steve. But he was young, only 51 years old. He seemed more forgetful, at times stumbling through sentences. They were more puzzled than concerned. Maybe it was just the normal "senior moments," they thought. But the symptoms worsened. By 2004, at the age of 54, Steve was diagnosed with early-onset Alzheimer's disease. For Mary and Steve, the diagnosis was life-altering: "The future, once rosy and full of promise, takes on a different set of colors, bleak and gray," wrote Dr. Newport of Steve's diagnosis. After the initial diagnosis, the disease progressed quickly. By 2008, "he was really going downhill. He was no longer driving and couldn't use a calculator [he was an accountant]."

Unwilling to give up, she dove into the research on Alzheimer's disease. Soon, a grim reality set in. Despite decades of research and billions of dollars spent, there was no viable treatment. Hundreds of drugs had shown promise only to fail in clinical trials. With no current treatment, she embraced the hope that something promising might be around the corner, and began searching for new clinical trials. Perhaps some emerging drug could help slow the disease, she hoped. Luck intervened. "There hadn't been any trials for several years in our area, and then two trials came along at the same time." With little to lose, Dr. Newport decided to have Steve screened for both trials.

The track record for Alzheimer's drugs to date was abysmal, some drugs with early promise were later found to accelerate the disease. Worried that these new drugs might do the same, she stayed up late into the night researching the risks and rewards of each candidate drug should Steve qualify for one or both trials. That evening, she stumbled onto a press release about a medical food that was expected to be available in about a years' time. That grabbed her attention. Two pilot studies had already been completed that tested this medical food with Alzheimer's patients. One study entered twenty patients and the other one hundred and fifty-two. In both studies, "they found that nearly half of the people with Alzheimer's who took this medical food had improved memory and cognition. You never hear that about Alzheimer's drugs," said Dr. Newport.

The press release didn't say what the medical food was, so she searched and found the patent application. It described a type of pathology in Alzheimer's that she had never heard of. "There is insulin resistance in the brain. It's like type 2 diabetes of the brain." The product contained a type of fat called medium-chain triglyceride (MCT) oil. As a neonatologist in the early 1980s, Dr. Newport recalled her use of MCT oil. "We used to put it directly into the feeding tube of our tiniest preemies." About that time, infant formula companies started adding MCT's in an attempt to mimic the fatty acid profile of breast milk, which contains 15 percent MCT's. The interesting thing about MCT oil, recalled Dr. Newport, was that it could cross the blood-brain barrier, enter neurons, and then skip over the normal regulatory transport of fats into cells to be directly processed into acetyl-coA. This caused the pool of acetyl-coA to spill over, thus leading to the enzymatic generation of ketones. This same process also occurs in the liver, releasing ketones in the circulation for other tissues to use. In that sense, MCT oil is a sort of "hack" to cheat your way into ketosis without fasting or a ketogenic diet. The patent then claimed that ketones had the ability to bypass the blockade from insulin resistance in the Alzheimer's brain and provide fuel for the starving brain.

At 9 a.m. the next morning, May 20, 2008, they arrived at the appointment that would determine if Steve would qualify for the first of two possible clinical trials. Steve would need to score a 16 out of 30 points on the Mini-Mental Status exam. "He only got 14 points that morning. We were heartbroken. The doctor asked him to draw a clock, it's a standard test for Alzheimer's and he drew several little circles and like four numbers, very random and not organized." Still reeling from Steve's performance in the exam, Dr. Newport remembered what she had read about the MCT-containing medical food the night before. With nothing to lose, she drove to the store to buy coconut oil (it contains 60% MCT). She did the math and calculated the quantities of coconut oil that corresponded to the amount of MCT given to the patients in the trials.

The next morning Steve was scheduled to go to the screening for the second clinical trial. Before they left, she gave him two tablespoons of coconut oil. "He gained 4 points from the day before, which is very significant. He knew what town we were in, he knew what floor we were on, what day of the week it was, and he remembered that it was spring, and those were things that he couldn't remember the day before."

Dr. Newport wondered if this striking improvement was simply good luck or if it was really due to the coconut oil. Realizing there was no harm in continuing, she started giving Steve coconut oil throughout the day. She noticed his cravings started to change. "He used to eat tons of fruit every night. Mangoes and grapes. I think his brain was starving and he was craving sugar." Slowly he stopped eating the fruit at night. And then he started leaving pasta, bread and rice on his plate. So I just started leaving it off."

Dr. Newport continued to research the connection between ketones and Alzheimer's, which led her to Dr. Veech. "We started talking," she recalled. "He was very interested in Steve's case." The improvements continued. "Steve used to have lots of trouble in the morning. He hardly talked, he couldn't figure out how to get water out of the refrigerator, couldn't figure out how to get a utensil out of the drawer, and he would have tremors when he tried to eat. That all went away within a couple of days. He was moving faster, he was talking again, whistling, the animation came back in his face. He told me 'it felt like a light switch had come on' in his brain the day he started the coconut oil."

Two weeks after starting the coconut oil, he was allowed to be rescreened for the first clinical trial. He was again asked to draw a clock. "This time it was a full circle with all the numbers and the hands," said Dr. Newport. At two months, his stiff, slow gait transformed back into a normal walk. He was able to tie his shoes again, which he had been unable to do for some time. And at four months he started reading again. "He had stopped reading for about a year and a half at that point. He was someone who read novels."

In the end, Steve ended up qualifying for both of the clinical trials. They chose the trial that consisted of an oral medication. The first year of the clinical trial, Dr. Newport could not be sure if his improvement was due to the coconut oil or the drug. "He improved so much that first year that he was able to start working as a volunteer at the hospital helping in the supply room," said Dr. Newport.

Once the trial was unblinded, they discovered something significant: he was on the placebo. This removed all doubt. Patients had been tested over the course of the trial to measure progress. The average score for the patients on the placebo was a loss of 6 points, where Steve had *gained* six points over the trial period.

For Dr. Newport, the revelation of Steve's remarkable progress due to something available at the local supermarket was overwhelming. "I felt like I had this really big secret that I had to tell the 36 million people in the world with Alzheimer's. I had to get this message out." So, she began writing. She wrote politicians, the media and Alzheimer's groups telling them about this medical food that was almost ready for release but that you could buy at the store now as coconut oil or a purified form of coconut oil that isolated the medium chain triglycerides. "To me it was criminal. And I was angry that I didn't know about this four years sooner," said Dr. Newport.

Dr. Newport's anger turned into action. She began attending conferences and telling Steve's story to anyone who would listen. She also kept up her conversations with Dr. Veech. He had explained that the ketone ester he was developing would be able to raise ketone levels ten times higher than MCT oil but that it was still in development. Eventually her advocacy efforts paid off. She started receiving invitations to speak at conferences and hospitals. The local newspaper picked up on it and wrote an article that included Dr. Veech. By 2009 the message was getting out to the people who needed to hear it the most. "Then I began to hear back from other people trying coconut and MCT oil," said Dr. Newport. Many people told her stories similar to Steve's: they, too, were seeing unexpected improvements. "I've collected over 500 emails from people. It's pretty dramatic," she said.

Sometime in mid-2009, still enrolled in the clinical trial, Steve got crossed over from the placebo to the active drug (crossing over is common in clinical trial design). They were still hopeful that the new drug might prove beneficial. Seven months after starting on the drug the side effects became unbearable and Dr. Newport had him stop taking it in March, 2010. Then, in the summer of 2010, they received a shocking phone call: the trial had been stopped because the data showed that the drug was *accelerating* the disease process. "March was right about the time that he started going downhill again," recalled Dr. Newport. She couldn't help but note the irony: the coconut oil, a cheap food she bought at the supermarket, led to improvements that allowed him to enter a clinical trial only to receive a drug that ended up accelerating the disease.

Through everything, she had maintained close contact with Dr. Veech. She called him and explained Steve's situation and that he had begun to decline again, most likely due to the drug. "You know, the toxicity testing has been completed on the ester, it looks really good," explained Veech. "He then asked if we wanted to be a clinical trial of one person," said Dr. Newport. "Of course, we said yes." A few days later a bottle of the ester showed up in the mail. "The very first dose Steve took, it was like the light bulb brightened up again. He had not been able to write the alphabet out at that point and it took him twenty minutes, but he did it. Twenty-four hours later, it turned him around."

"He was very stable for the next twenty months," said Dr. Newport. "He was much happier and again regained the ability to do tasks and be autonomous. We were very grateful to Dr. Veech." It is extremely rare for Alzheimer's patients to improve over time. Although anecdotal, considering Alzheimer's patients almost never improve, Dr. Newport and Dr. Veech felt it was worth publishing Steve's experience as a case report presenting the results over the course of his 20 months on the ester. The abstract summarized Steve's experience: "The patient improved markedly in mood, affect, self-care, and cognitive and daily activity performance. The KME (ketone ester) was well tolerated throughout the 20-month treatment period. Cognitive performance tracked plasma -hydroxybutyrate concentrations, with noticeable improvements in conversation and interaction at the higher levels, compared with pre-dose levels."

Steve remained on the ester until a terrible accident occurred in 2013. He fell backwards, hitting his head sharply. "He was still doing very well when he fell, still able to do the tasks he couldn't do when he was diagnosed," said Dr. Newport. The fall triggered a massive seizure. "He never recovered from that." The trauma was too much and precipitated a rapid decline, ultimately leading to his death in January of 2016.

Dr. Newport can't help but reflect on the timing. For Alzheimer's patients like Steve, prevention or early treatment may end up being the critical variable. "Steve was far into the disease process when he started the ester. I think that if we could have gotten the ester early on it would have made a huge difference. I think this therapy has incredible potential for prevention."

By the time of Steve's death in 2016, the environment surrounding ketosis had changed dramatically. Gary Taubes struck again, publishing *Good Calories Bad Calories* in 2007, making a compelling case that a high-fat, low-carbohydrate was, in fact, a healthier way of eating. The ketogenic diet, once lost to the history books, was being resurrected by popular media health advocates for its ability to reduce weight, improve general health, and provide mental clarity. Dominic D'Agostino, a ketone researcher at the University of South Florida, bridged the gap between the research and the mounting appetite of the popular media. D'Agostino, both charismatic and knowledgeable, extolled the virtues of the ketogenic diet in articles, interviews, TED talks, and podcasts, including the far-reaching Joe Rogan Experience, with 190 million downloads per month.

The awareness within the neurological community continued to grow. Veech published two studies showing significant improvement when comparing outcomes in mice fed the ketone ester compared to a standard high-carbohydrate control diet. When mice engineered to develop a neurodegenerative disease similar to Alzheimer's were fed the ester, they behaved more normally, retained better memories and exploratory behavior, and had significantly less neurofibrillary tangles and amyloid plaques than the mice eating the standard mouse chow. A 2009 randomized, double-blind, placebo-controlled trial of 152 mild-to-moderate Alzheimer's patients given MCT oil resulted in "significant" improvement in cognitive scores compared to placebo. In 2018, a randomized, controlled trial with 47 Parkinson's patients compared a high-carbohydrate/low-fat diet to a ketogenic diet. While both groups improved, the ketogenic diet group showed strikingly more improvement. Compared to baseline, test scores in the ketogenic diet group improved 41 percent while scores in the high-carbohydrate, low-fat group improved by only 11 percent. A 2006 study published in the *Lancet* using mice bred to develop ALS, showed that mice fed a ketogenic diet had significantly higher motor performance and motor neuron counts when compared to the control mice. Another study showed the ketogenic diet reduced cerebral edema and improved cerebral metabolism and behavioral outcomes in rodents subjected to traumatic brain injuries. "Ketosis has the potential to treat *all* of the neurodegenerative diseases," says Dr. Newport. Today her message resonates across the globe and she has trouble keeping up with demand. "This year I was scheduled to give talks in Germany, Singapore, and various states in the United States, but then the virus (COVID-19) hit."

The growing popularity spilled over into other medical research, too. A maverick researcher from Boston College, Thomas Seyfried, published the 2012 book, *Cancer as a Metabolic Disease*, reexamining the 1924 claim from Otto Warburg that "the prime cause of cancer is the replacement of the respiration of oxygen in normal body cells by a fermentation of sugar." Translated: cancer cells tend to rely less on oxidative phosphorylation (the electron transport chain) and more on *aerobic glycolysis*—generating energy using glucose and the glycolytic pathway and kicking out the end product lactate, even in the presence of oxygen. Seyfried compiled an impressive body of evidence suggesting the ketogenic diet might be a viable therapy for cancer, targeting the metabolic dysfunction of the cancer cell that Warburg had observed almost a century before.

Subsequent clinical trials proved the safety of the diet and enhanced survival in cancer patients. A review article published in 2020 titled "Ketogenic Diet in the Treatment of Cancer: Where do We Stand?" tallied the evidence from dozens of preclinical studies and dozens of clinical trials and concluded that "the ketogenic diet probably creates an unfavorable metabolic environment for cancer cells and thus can be regarded as a promising adjuvant as a patient-specific multifactorial therapy." For cancer, the ketogenic diet has been shown to have an exquisitely targeted effect. Specifically, cancer cells have trouble burning ketones efficiently while normal cells do not. The upshot is that cancer cells have a less efficient antioxidant system under ketosis while healthy cells have a more efficient antioxidant system. Because most cancer therapies are oxidative (kill cancer cells by inducing free radicals), this sets up a *therapeutic differential* where cancer cells are more easily killed and healthy cells are better equipped to withstand the toxic effects of chemotherapy and radiation. A small trial showed that a simple 48-72-hour ketosis-inducing fast immediately before chemotherapy dramatically reduced the corrosive side-effects from radiation and chemotherapy. A more recent randomized phase 2 trial testing a "fasting-mimicking diet" combined with chemotherapy resulted in a 300-400 percent increase in the chance of killing 90-100 percent of cancer cells in women with breast cancer. "The results suggest that an FMD [fasting-mimicking diet] significantly reinforces the effects of neoadjuvant chemotherapy on the radiological and pathological tumor response in patients with HER2 negative early breast cancer," wrote the authors of the study. Moreover, there was less DNA damage in T-cells in patients who received the FMD with chemotherapy.

The resurgence of the ketogenic diet offered new hope for type 2 diabetes patients as well. Globally, type 2 diabetes is a rapidly evolving health crisis. Today, the majority of adults in the United States (52.3%) have either type 2 diabetes (14.3%) or prediabetes (38%), a category that hovers just a hop, skip and a jump away from full-blown type 2 diabetes. The cost of treating type 2 diabetes in the United States is staggering: over $240 billion per year, and rising at a dizzying rate. Again, the progression of prediabetes to diabetes is intimately tied to insulin resistance—the decreasing ability of the cellular machinery to shuttle glucose into the cell and then process it through glycolysis → Krebs cycle → electron transport chain. The metabolic dysfunction of insulin resistance causes glucose to linger in the bloodstream. Glucose is a rigid, planer molecule that physically damages the tissues it comes in close and continued contact with. With the failure of insulin to clear glucose from circulation, people with diabetes can expect to experience a domino-like series of devastating health conditions, from nerve damage and cardiovascular disease to kidney disease, blindness, impotence, weight gain, brain fog, and critically—considering the viral pandemic we currently face—a poorly functioning immune system.

Veech and Cahill showed that ketosis elegantly sidesteps the pathological blockades imposed by insulin resistance. In 2014 a team of forward-thinking entrepreneurs realized that a carefully implemented program, delivered remotely, could educate people with diabetes in how to eat a ketogenic diet, then track their markers and support their compliance. The company, called Virta Health, began offering this drugless treatment to people with diabetes in 2014. So far, the results have been remarkable. Sixty percent of the patients on the ketogenic diet reversed their type 2 diabetes over the course of a year. The patients eliminated 63 percent of diabetes-specific medications and 94 percent of patients eliminated or reduced insulin usage. On average, the patients lost 30 lbs each and had dramatic improvements in inflammation markers, lipid profiles, blood pressure and a 12 percent relative reduction in 10-year atherosclerotic cardiovascular disease risk score. *All from simply reducing the amount of carbohydrate they ate.*

With regard to the original DARPA mission to improve the endurance of warfighters, whispers of a new ketone ester being developed as a potential performance enhancer trickled into the competitive cycling community where riders are always searching for any sort of competitive advantage. In the 2012 Summer Olympics, the British team dominated cycling with 12 medals, eight of them gold. Many reports suggested that it was no coincidence that Clarke, at Oxford, was simultaneously developing the ester (It was formally released to the public in 2018 with the formation of two new companies, HVMN and KetoneAid). Years later, Clarke confirmed the rumors: "They were first used in 2012 at the Tour de France and then the London Olympics," said Clarke. "We'd bottle them up and hand deliver them. The team who used them at the Tour drank one bottle before, during and straight after the stage, plus in the evening."

In 2016, Veech and Clarke published a study showing that highly-trained cyclists were able to improve their performance in a 30-minute time trial by 2 percent after ingesting the ketone ester. Two percent may not sound like a lot, but in a sport like cycling it is a colossal advantage. The Tour de France is often decided by a few minutes after 28 days of racing—a fraction of a percent.

By 2018 the cat was out of the bag. The CEO of HVMN, Geoff Woo, was reported in *Telegraph Sports* saying that "Seven teams were buying the ester from his company in preparation for the Tour de France. I know a couple of riders who, instead of buying it through their teams, are buying it personally to make sure they don't run out of stock. We've worked with a few cyclists who are looking to break the hour record. Top-level cyclists. We've sold $200,000 worth of stock in the last few months just to cycling teams alone." In the 2019 Tour de France team Jumbo-Visma jumped off to a dominating start, winning four stages early on in the race. Later the team manager confirmed their use of ketones to Dutch newspaper *De Telegraaf*, calling the ester a "miracle drink."

Cyclists were now claiming the ester gave them a decided advantage—especially in grueling stage-races like the Tour de France—claiming it not only improved performance, but also granted an "unprecedented" ability to recover—often the deciding factor in races of attrition like the Tour de France. A 2019 study confirmed the experience of the cyclists. The study had the subjects participate in an intense three-week-long training camp to simulate a competition like the Tour de France. Nine subjects consumed a ketone ester and nine others took a placebo. The test group drank up to three 25 g doses of the ketone ester [96% (R)-3-hydroxybutyl (R)-3-hydroxybutyrate] per day, one immediately after each workout (2 workouts per day) and one before going to bed. By the third week of the camp, the group that consumed the ketones was able to perform a sustained training load an eye-popping 15 percent higher than the placebo group, including a power output that was 15 percent higher in a time trial. At the end of these three weeks, the cyclists in both groups had a reduction in their max heart rate during maximal and submaximal exercise, which is typical following a long period of intense training. However, the reduction in heart rate was more pronounced in subjects who consumed the ketone supplement, suggesting a profound effect of the ester on recovery.

The ability of ketone supplementation appears to extend beyond physiological performance. A study performed in the fall of 2018 demonstrated a remarkable ability of the ester to sustain cognitive function in athletes as well. The double-blind, randomized trial had eleven male soccer players take a cognitive test battery, run until exhaustion, and then again take the same cognitive test.

A carbohydrate-electrolyte solution was consumed before and during exercise either alone or with an amount of ketone ester that resulted in blood BHB levels of 1.5 to 2.6 mM during exercise. The results were striking. "I was amazed that the ketone ester group had the same exact scores as the start of the performance. Meanwhile the placebo group had double the wrong answers. This is like a 4th quarter quarterback having the sharpness of the 1st quarter," said Frank Llosa, the CEO of KetoneAid.

With the twenty first century in full swing, the explosion in studies looking beyond athletic performance has demonstrated the unique ability of ketosis to treat a sweeping spectrum of life-altering diseases; Veech and Cahill's 2001 prediction that ketosis could treat a list that "would encompass almost every disease state" was proving remarkably insightful. In particular, ketosis seems to concentrate its therapeutic effect in the brain. Study after study suggests a potent therapeutic effect countering the corrosive effect of insulin resistance on the aging brain. And with over half of the US adult population suffering from prediabetes or frank diabetes, the consequences are enormous. Indeed, Warburg, Krebs and Veech had a visceral desire to gain a deeper understanding of the diseases that were poorly understood at the time—diseases with no viable treatments that affected a massive swath of the population—diseases like Alzheimer's and dementia (at present,

30 percent of people are expected to develop dementia). Poetically, this thread of desire, reaching back through history and passed from Warburg to Krebs to Veech, culminated in a promising therapy to prevent the pernicious and relentless progression of cognitive decline.

Let's walk through a scenario illustrating the power of ketones to affect brain health as we "naturally" age. A typical person in American in their 40s has most likely already begun to develop some degree of insulin resistance. What this means for the brain is that it is not getting the energy it needs to function efficiently as glucose uptake in neurons becomes more and more restricted. Stephen Cunnane, a researcher at Sherbrook University in Canada, describes this developing scenario as an "energy gap" between the brain's high energy demands met by an inadequate supply. Past the age of sixty-five, even healthy adults with no other problems have developed a "brain energy gap" of 14 percent on average. For people with a genetic predisposition for Alzheimer's and diabetes this gap develops much earlier, and in people with early-onset Alzheimer's the gap widens to 30 percent. "Anybody trying to function with 20 percent less brain glucose long term will suffer from brain exhaustion," said Cunnane. By the time someone develops full-blown Alzheimer's disease the energy gap has expanded to 40 percent. The brain of the Alzheimer's patient is starving. "We believe that this energy gap increases the risk of neuronal dysfunction and cognitive decline," says Cunnane. The brain, unable to charge the nucleotide coenzymes like ATP, as Veech showed, all metabolic processes suffer. And according to Cunnane, this precipitates damage to neurons and a cascading decline in cognition.

The emergence of this energy gap is linked to our metabolic health. In those who eat a standard American diet and engage in little activity, it rears its ugly head far too early in life. Cunnane's research clearly shows that the gap is apparent in PET scans long before the first symptoms appear. As the gap widens, symptoms appear but are written off as "senior moments" or "normal" forgetfulness. Emergence or worsening of fatigue, apathy, depression, and other cognitive related issues are too readily accepted as a "normal" part of the aging process. The most recent study by Veech used MRI scans to visualize this erosion of cognitive functionality as the brain is starved of energy. The study focused on "brain networks," the connections between different regions of the brain that promote coordinated cognition. The stability of these networks is critical to higher-level cognitive function. As these networks break down, the coordinated flow of neural impulses from one area of the brain to another becomes impaired, much like a breakdown in traffic signals at a handful of busy intersections can snarl the smooth flow of traffic, causing gridlock citywide. The study showed that critically important brain networks have already begun to break down by the age of 47, and that this "destabilization correlates with poorer cognition and accelerates with insulin resistance."

Ketones promise a solution. By skirting the glycolytic pathway and entering the Krebs cycle directly, ketones bypass all the barriers of insulin resistance. Critically, they offer an alternative fuel to *fill* the energy gap and restore smooth signaling in the brain's networks. Veech compared the scans of subjects on a standard diet to subjects on a ketogenic diet after fasting in order to measure the direct impact of different fuel sources. They had the subjects in both groups fast overnight and then ingest a drink containing equal amounts of calories from either glucose or ketone ester. The subjects eating a ketogenic diet and ingesting the ester showed brain networks had stabilized. In contrast, the subjects on the standard diet and ingesting glucose showed a destabilization of brain networks.

This is no trivial matter. Cognitive decline, whether from Alzheimer's, dementia, or even what we consider "normal" aging robs millions of people every year of the ability to function optimally. It robs them of self-reliance and the ability to enjoy life to the fullest. Like a slow lowering of a curtain blocking sunlight, emotions are muted, memories fade, and apathy takes over. Ketone metabolism, whether it comes from a ketogenic diet, periodic fasting, exogenous ketones, or a combination of sources, holds the promise to mitigate this decline in brain health that impacts so many lives. We just have to muster the motivation to be proactive in a health care system and economy that is primarily reactive. "Intellectuals solve problems, geniuses prevent them," said Einstein.

"IT'S THE KETONES, STUPID"

K etone metabolism, we now know, is much more than just an extraordinarily efficient auxiliary motor that kicks in during bouts of food deprivation. The potent ability of ketosis to prevent or slow a range of disease processes alludes to a *deeper* purpose. Food deprivation, known as *calorie restriction*, has proven to be the only way to consistently increase the lifespan across all eukaryotic (multicellular) species, from yeast and round-worms to fruit flies and monkeys. The phenomenon is far too ubiquitous to be a coincidence, and, evolutionarily, it makes intuitive, Darwinian sense. When food was unavailable, extending lifespan would increase the probability of making it to the other side of the famine when enough resources were once again available improving the odds of reproduction.

The lifespan-increasing power of caloric restriction was first observed in 1935 by scientists at Cornell University. Clive McCay and his colleagues put rats on a very low-calorie diet and extended the animals' maximal lifespan by an astonishing 30 to 50 percent. McCay couldn't say why caloric restriction worked, just that it *did* work. Clearly, McCay realized caloric restriction was slowing the aging process, but no one knew *how*, or, for that matter, *why* multicellular organisms age in the first place.

Hundreds of theories on aging were proposed over the twentieth century but the only one that withstood the test of time was a theory proposed by Denham Harman at the University of Nebraska Medical Center. Harman's theory, called the Free Radical Theory of Aging, proposed that the damage to cellular structures from the inevitable leakage of free radicals from the electron transport chain was the ultimate cause of aging. The theory made two predictions. Number one, if free radicals are the cause of aging, then antioxidants, the molecules that neutralize them, should extend lifespan. And number two, the damage from free radicals should accumulate over time, especially in the mitochondrial DNA. Mitochondrial DNA should take the brunt of the damage, predicted Harmon, due to simple proximity. The mitochondrial DNA sits defenseless immediately adjacent to the electron transport chain—the source of free radicals. It's like putting critical information on a DVD and then storing it in the oven—eventually someone is going to turn on the oven and damage the DVD. Due to this odd placement, mitochondrial DNA undergoes mutations at a rate 100,000 times than that of DNA in the nucleus.

Yet, Harmon's two predictions confounded a generation of biologists. It didn't mean his theory was necessarily wrong, but it did need rethinking from its original form. The first prediction, that antioxidants should extend life, was tested for decades; no matter which antioxidants were used in which dose, it didn't matter—they simply didn't extend life. "By the 1990s it was clear that antioxidants are not a panacea for ageing and disease, and only fringe medicine still peddles this notion," wrote an expert in the field. Second, the prediction that mitochondrial DNA mutations should accumulate as we age also proved to be untrue. No matter how hard researchers looked, the mutations in the protein coding regions of the thirteen mitochondrial genes were found in just a tiny fraction of cells, hardly enough to account for the profound functional decline that occurs during the aging process.

Researchers offered up two explanations for this strange state of affairs. Number one, perhaps antioxidants needed to be targeted to the mitochondria—the actual source of the free radical damage—to have an effect. Second, maybe the reason researchers were unable to find the mitochondrial DNA mutations was that other vital cellular processes dispose of mitochondria with mutated DNA.

Remember, each cell has many hundreds of mitochondria. So, if a single mitochondrion experiences catastrophic damage to its DNA, it will be unable to manufacture functional proteins for the electron transport chain complexes, and the electron transport chain will grind to a sudden halt. This causes the mitochondrial membrane potential to collapse and the mitochondrion is then broken down and recycled. In this scenario, the mutation is removed from the mitochondrial pool. But imagine another scenario where a less catastrophic mutation occurs that results in a still-functional yet defective electron transport chain complex. This manifests in a still operational but slightly less efficient electron transport chain. Over time, the mutated mitochondrion reproduces and the cell becomes less and less efficient at generating energy as it is burdened with more and more of these defective mitochondria. The upshot of this scenario is that ATP becomes progressively less "charged" and once a threshold level is reached, energy sensors are tripped and an exquisitely evolved self-disposal system called *apoptosis* is activated. Apoptosis is rightfully nicknamed "programed cell death," an altruistic act of self-sacrifice intended to preserve the health of the organism—part of the fine print in the contract that was written and signed eons ago between single-cellular life allowing it to evolve into multicellular life. Apoptosis would explain why researchers can't find an accumulation of even subtle mutations to mitochondrial DNA. Multicellular organisms are just very good at getting rid of them.

One would be forgiven, then, for wondering why we age at all. If the body has evolved extraordinary and efficient systems to dispose of the damage from free radicals—the main source of cellular damage—then why do we experience the functional decline known as aging? The reason appears to center on stem cells.

Hidden in niches throughout the body reservoirs of stem cells stand ready to replace lost cells. Indeed, it is easy to notice that the human body is a machine like no other—renewing from the inside out—a machine with an intrinsic capacity to *fix itself*. "The body concentrates order. It continuously self-repairs. Every five days you get a new stomach lining. You get a new liver every two months. Your skin replaces itself every six weeks. Every year, 98 percent of the atoms of your body are replaced," wrote evolutionary biologist Lynn Margulis.

For every cell that undergoes apoptosis—about 50 billion per day—a stem cell must divide to replace it. This happens efficiently when we are young, with stem cells perfectly balancing cells lost to apoptosis. However, as we age stem cells experience a functional decline known as a loss of "stemness" and the balance tips more toward apoptosis than renewal. More cells are dying than are being replaced. This is why older adults shrink and their organs weigh substantially less compared to when they were young. After age 40, the volume of the brain and/or its weight declines with age at a rate of around 5 percent per decade. This then begs the question: Why do stem cells lose the ability to repair as we age? The answer to this question comes from a fascinating new theory proposed by David Sinclair at Harvard, called the Informational Theory of Aging.

Sinclair's theory hinges on an exploding branch of biology called *epigenetics*. In the 1940s Nobel Prize winning physicist Edwin Schrodinger wrote a book titled *What is Life?* Life, claimed Schrodinger, is fundamentally *information*. He imagined the cell to contain some sort of "code-script" that imparted all of the majestic functionality of life. Schrodinger's eerily accurate prediction was validated in 1953 with the famous discovery of DNA's structure by Watson and Crick. The same year that Schrodinger made his proclamation an English embryologist named Conrad Waddington coined the word *epigenetics*. "Epi" is Greek for "above" or "on." Epigenetics is cellular function "above" traditional genetics. And this description is not metaphorical. It is physical. With little evidence, Waddington made the bold claim that epigenetics was the more "interesting" branch of genetics. In other words, epigenetics accounted for *most* of the "information" that defined multicellular life. Genes were "single stamps," said Waddington. What was far more interesting for Waddington was a "conceptual album to put them in." What he meant was this: the 20,000 genes in our genome are like a computer's binary code, 1s and 0s. By itself, binary code is meaningless. It is the next level of organization that derives the meaning—a sea of 1s and 0s combining to form programs like artificial intelligence, for example.

When Watson and Crick unveiled the structure of DNA to the world the field of epigenetics was pushed far to the periphery. With few researchers interested in the exiled field it took decades to sort out the mechanics behind the epigenetic code. The word *code* is an abstraction, yet it is grounded in *material*. DNA does not exist alone, it is mixed up with protein into a complex called *chromatin*. In the late eighteenth century, a German biochemist named Albrecht Kossel discovered that chromatin contains an interesting repeating protein that is attached to DNA. Kossel named this repeating unit a *histone*. In the decades that followed histones became the focus of an intense curiosity. For most of the twentieth century geneticists and biochemists were puzzled by their role in chromatin. Researchers knew histones were globally bound to DNA, huddling together in every bend, fold, corner and cleft, but their purpose remained unclear. This intimate association with DNA seduced researchers into speculating that histones were involved in the regulation of genetic expression, but the precise mechanism remained elusive. "Because of the close association of histones with DNA in the cells of higher organisms," wrote a biophysicist in 1969. "it has been suggested that histones are involved in genetic regulation and much effort has been expended in attempting to demonstrate this role. However, histones are a major component of chromosomes and they could be involved in a purely structural role"

The "structural role" of histones quickly became apparent. From a physical standpoint, histones appeared as evolution's solution to a packaging problem—packaging up the massive amount of DNA multicellular organism tote from one generation to the next. Within each one of our 40 trillion cells, our 46 chromosomes stretched end to end comprise about three meters of DNA. Clearly evolution had to come up with a solution to package our chromosomal luggage into the vanishingly small volume of the nucleus, a space one millionth of an inch across.

Histones solved this problem. They are globular, ball-shaped proteins with a single amino acid tail dangling outward that wind DNA up like thread on a spool, condensing it into a fiber that then coils upon itself repeatedly, forming "supercoiled" loops (coils upon coils). Perhaps histones *were* nothing more than inert packaging molecules. Nothing more than "the biochemical equivalent of nuts, bolts, and bungee cords to keep the all-important genetic molecule in its proper dimensions," with all the charm, as one researcher put it, "of a brick wall."

But then a flurry of papers in 1996 by a biochemist named Davis Allis at Rockefeller University in New York, all-at-once shattered the notion histones were little more than a boring packaging protein. Allis illuminated histones as a centerpiece of dynamic epigenetic regulation. Specifically, Allis discovered a class of enzymes called a *histone acetyltransferases*, or HATs for short. Allis discovered that HATs "turn up" genes. To accomplish this, HATs attach an acetyl group (2-carbon group) to the tail of the histones surrounding the gene to be upregulated. The attached acetyl group then neutralizes the positive charge of certain amino acids in the histone, thus reducing the attraction between histones and the slightly negatively charged DNA—loosening the nuts, and undoing the bungee cords—relaxing the hyper-condensed coils of chromatin and making it easier for RNA polymerase to transcribe the associated gene.

If the cell had a positive regulator of gene expression in the form of HATs, perhaps, reasoned Allis, they also had a negative regulator. A negative regulator—an *anti-HAT*—realized Allis, would allow gene expression to operate like a toggle switch—genes could be actively turned up and down. A month later Allis isolated the anti-HAT enzymes. The enzymes, called *histone deacetylases*, removed the acetyl groups that HATs attached. Essentially, Allis had elucidated a new layer of *control* within the epigenome. HATs were pencils, writing instructions to turn up the expression of genes, and histone deacetylases were the erasers. "It couldn't have been a more wonderful one-two punch. I am not sure the chromatin field has been the same since," said Allis. "It wasn't rocket science to figure out this enzyme pair of reactions might function as an on/off switch . . . you couldn't turn your back on what these findings were saying. Most people thought chromatin was just a passive platform that wraps the DNA. But those two papers made people think about a more active process in which chromatin truly participates."

In the years that followed, additional histone "tags" were identified. Investigators revealed that histones appeared like Christmas trees—adorned with a rich diversity of "ornaments" that regulate gene expression. These chemical "ornaments" that embroider the tails of histones represented a new biological language. Collectively, the "ornaments"—and the lavishly complicated new level of regulation they occupied—became known as the *histone code*. Since Allis's first volley of papers in 1996, over 50 different histone modifications have been discovered. Taken together, the rich diversity of the histone code is able to smooth-out gene expression with far more control than a simple on/off toggle switch—transmitting incremental signals that control gene expression more like volume control dials.

For the entire twentieth century epigenetics had taken a back seat to traditional genetics, but with Allis's 1996 discovery the field of epigenetics found a foothold and leapt forward. The millennium marked the transition. "Epigeneticists, once a subcaste of biologist nudged to the far peripheries of the discipline now find themselves firmly at its epicenter," wrote Pulitzer Prize-winning author Siddhartha Mukherjee. The central reason for this transition was the growing realization that traditional genetics had failed miserably in answering the most compelling questions in biology: *What* makes us different? *Why* is someone tall and someone else short? *Why* does one person develop a disease and another does not?

It was always assumed that the genetic code—or more specifically—the *variation* in the genetic code from one person to another, would answer these fundamental questions. Yet once DNA sequencing technology progressed to where individual genomes could be sequenced and compared, researchers were stunned by the "lack" of diversity from one person's genome to the next. In short, our genomes are remarkably similar, far too similar to explain the variation in traits and disease from one person to the next. "Our DNA is overwhelmingly identical. Indeed, all of the beautiful permutations of the human form—the differences between the tallest and the shortest, the brown-eyed and the green eyed—are explained by just a tiny fraction of those base-pairs . . . finding the genetic differences that make one person taller or shorter than another is like looking for needles in a haystack," wrote science reporter Brian Resnick.

Waddington had been right all along—the epigenome was proving to be far more interesting and important than the fixed-code of the genome—and offered explanations where the genome failed. Genes are like plumbing parts that we share with other species: pipes, caps, elbows and splices that each species assembles in their own unique way. And truth be told, genes have a limited capacity to evolve, they wear an evolutionary straight jacket of sorts. Once a protein evolves to perform a certain function, like hemoglobin for example, it's capacity to evolve further is limited. The corollary to this is everywhere around us. Once an airplane wing was perfected, for example, i was difficult to perfect it further. Bats, which are mammals, evolved wings separately from birds, yet they still *look* like bird wings—evolution is limited by the number of engineering solutions that exist to solve a problem. It is the same with genes. We share 50 percent of our genes with a banana, 70 percent with single-celled yeast, 85 percent with a mouse, and our genome is almost identical to that of a chimpanzee.

To clarify the difference between epigenetics and genetics think of it this way: your genome is the *hardware*—the fixed genetic script you inherit from your mother and father. And your epigenome is the *software*, the programming responsible for turning the volume dials on all 20,000 of your genes. If DNA is a piano, then your epigenome is the pianist. Epigenetics is the music of life.

Epigenetics accounts for the remarkable division of labor found in multicellular life. All forty trillion cells in your body contain the exact same 46 chromosomes, yet the expression of genes is different from one cell type to the next. A liver cell, for example, has liver-related genes turned on, and the genes to manufacture stomach acid turned off. Epigenetics is also responsible for the awe-inspiring process of *embryogenesis*—the intrinsic program tripped by fertilization that directs the cascade of events marshaling a single celled zygote to a fully formed multi-cellular organism. Moreover, it is the epigenome that *alone* determines the complexity of an organism. Consider this: we have about the same number of genes as the 959-celled microscopic worm called C. *elegans*, roughly 20,000, yet our rich epigenome is what sets us apart. C. *elegans* can only play chopsticks on its piano, where we can play Mozart. "Nature," wrote Conrad Waddington, "is more like an artist than an engineer."

Now we know that in addition to accounting for most of the diversity *within* species, and the complexity *between* species, the epigenome accounts for the development of most diseases too. Very few diseases have an exclusively genetic origin, most are an amalgam of genetics and epi-genetics. Identical twins provide powerful evidence for this. Identical twins have the exact same genetic script, yet they rarely die of the same disease. This observation alone forced scientists back to the age-old question of nature ver-sus nurture: Which biological force has the majority influ-ence over our destiny? To clarify: our inherited genome is *nature*, the code we are handed. And our epigenomes operate through *nurture*, the effervescent and intangible environmental signals like trauma, triumph, loneliness, victories and love. And more tangible signals like nutri-tional inputs, exercise and toxins. Inside the epigenome, these inputs are calculated daily. Genes are turned up and turned down moment to moment. The output of this vast and fluctuation algorithm influences our moods, colors our thinking, and governs the innermost workings of our body on a molecular level. When this equation is all tallied up, the influence of nature accounts for about 20 percent of our longevity. Nurture, however, acting through the flexible and dynamic epigenome, accounts for *80 percent*. The chiseling and sculpting that life imposes on our epig-enome has the majority influence on how long we live. "Genes are not our destiny," said a leading expert in the field.

Yet the epigenome is designed to fail. Unlike the fixed code of our genome, the installed information within the epigenome "drifts" as we age. We are born with a freshly installed operating system—when we are conceived our epigenomes are wiped clean and installed anew. But over time, the sharp fidelity of our epigenome begins to fade. The main reason for this is damage to nuclear DNA. This is where Sinclair's Informational Theory of Aging unites with Harmon's Free Radical Theory of Aging.

In addition to wreaking all sorts of havoc on mito-chondrial DNA, free radicals also damage nuclear DNA in an assortment of different ways. The cell, however, has evolved exquisite mechanisms that attempt to repair this damage before there is a catastrophic system failure triggering apoptosis. Research has shown that a class of proteins called sirtuins are integral to the DNA repair process. Yet, strangely, sirtuins evolved to perform another critically important task: maintaining the integrity of the epigenome. Sirtuins are found scattered throughout the nucleus directing the attachment of the "ornaments" that adjust the dials on all 20,000 genes to just the right posi-tion. In other words, sirtuins keep the pianist playing beautiful music. Giving sirtuins two critically important jobs almost seems like evolution set them up to fail.

Here is how they fail: when there is damage to DNA, sirtuins are recruited to the site of the damage to help in the repair process. Once the DNA is repaired, the sirtuins then travel back to their original positions in the genome to restore the fidelity of the epigenome. But Sinclair dis-covered this process is not perfect. Sometimes, after a DNA repair event, the sirtuins don't make it back to their exact original location. This results in misplaced "ornaments" to histones and slightly different gene expression. Over time these errors add up, resulting in more pronounced misexpression of genes. Genes get inappropriately turned up or down and cells begin to lose their Identity. "A cell's identity changes. A skin cell starts behaving differently, turning on genes that were shut off in the womb and were meant to stay off. Now it is 90 percent a skin cell and 10 percent other cell types, all mixed up, with properties of neurons and kidney cells. The cell becomes inept at the things skin cells must do, such as making hair, keeping the skin supple, and healing when injured," said Sinclair.

Sinclair's laboratory has compiled compelling evidence that this movement of sirtuins, to and from the site of DNA damage, leads to the epigenetic "drift" behind aging. In a brilliant experiment, Sinclair showed that repeatedly damaging the DNA in mice—even though the damage was repaired perfectly by the DNA repair enzymes—results in sirtuins misplacing some of the "ornaments" on histones that dictate gene expression. The pianist begins to miss keys and play out of tune, and the mice age much faster, *50% faster*. This loss of epigenetic "information" is the underpinning of the Informational Theory of Aging. Genes that should remain quiet get turned on, and other genes get turned down or off inappropriately—once pristine cells began to function poorly. "Here's the vital takeaway," says Sinclair. "We could age mice without affecting any of the most commonly assumed causes of aging. We hadn't made their cells mutate. We hadn't touched their telomeres. We hadn't messed with their mitochondria. We hadn't directly exhausted their stem cells. Yet the mice were suffering from a loss of body mass, mitochondria, and muscle strength and an increase in cataracts, arthritis, dementia, bone loss, and frailty. All of the symptoms of aging—the conditions that push mice, like humans, farther toward the precipice of death—were being caused not by mutation but by the epigenetic changes that come as a result of DNA damage signals. We hadn't given the mice all of those ailments. We had given them aging."

Here's the important point: this pernicious process of epigenetic drift affects all cells, *yet seems to particularly affect the function of stem cells negatively.* The consequence of stem cells losing their epigenetic programming is a diminished capacity to replace the cells lost to apoptosis. Loss without renewal. The perfect storm.

This model of aging suggests a two-pronged approach to slowing the process: first, slow the main source of damage—free radical production. And second, help sirtuins to do both of their jobs: repairing DNA damage *and* preserving the epigenome thus allowing stem cells to maintain their critical functionality. In other words, mitigating the damage that leads to cell loss from apoptosis and/or preserving the ability of stem cells to replace lost cells by maintaining the epigenome should theoretically slow the aging process.

Extrapolating from its time-tested ability to extend life, caloric restriction must be accomplishing one or both of those tasks. Veech firmly believed that the life-extending

benefits of caloric restriction weren't really that complicated. He believed it was due to production of ketones
induced by restricting calories—more specifically, largely
due to beta-hydroxybutyrate itself. "It's the beta-hydroxybutyrate stupid," he would say jokingly, when explaining
the effects of caloric restriction to others. Indeed, Veech's
research had uncovered an astonishing property of BHB
that strikes at the heart of the source of the damage
behind aging: a dramatic reduction in endogenous free
radical production. Endogenous free radical production
is unavoidable—like Harmon noted in the 50s—they are
an inevitable byproduct of normal metabolism. Stripping
electrons from NADH and whipping them through a
series of cytochrome complexes inexorably results in some
escaping. Most of the naturally produced free radicals in
the cell come from the mitochondrial coenzyme Q couple. Electrons tend to linger on the coenzyme Q couple as
they are transported down the electron transport chain.
The upshot of this "lingering" is that some free radicals
escape. One of the most striking manifestations of ketosis that Veech uncovered was the oxidation of the coenzyme Q couple. Recall that oxidation means *less* electrons.
During ketosis, as electrons are passed down the chain,
they don't linger as long. Consequently, *dramatically* fewer
free radicals are produced.

Moreover, glutathione, the cell's "master antioxidant,"
is powered by NADPH. Because BHB charges NADPH
further, glutathione is recycled faster, transitioning more
quickly back to its antioxidant form, allowing it to mop

up free radicals more efficiently—like a vacuum with a faster spinning brush. The media has saturated us with the importance of antioxidants to overall health. Yet the message surrounding antioxidants is in strange discordance with the science. We are continuously told to eat foods and even take supplements that contain antioxidants, yet Krebs and Veech long ago established that consuming antioxidants didn't even make a bit of difference in the cells' ability to neutralize free radicals—the antioxidant potential of the cell was dictated solely by the ratio of NADPH to NADP. "It used to drive Veech crazy when people extolled the virtues of ingesting antioxidants like vitamin C or polyphenols," said a colleague. "You can't change the redox state by feeding antioxidants," said Veech. "The only way you can control the redox state, the only way I know was with ketosis . . . All these other reducing agents [antioxidants] are nonsense." Krebs even admonished the great Linus Pauling who recommended massive quantities of vitamin C in part, because he thought it was a potent antioxidant. "Please quit lying about what you do not understand," Krebs wrote to Pauling. The reason that ingesting large amounts of molecular antioxidants like vitamin C don't increase the neutralization of free radicals is because every time vitamin C neutralizes a free radical it becomes oxidized and *must* be recycled back to its reduced form to neutralize another free radical, and the only way it can be recycled back to its reduced form is by NADPH. Therefore, increasing the "pool" of intracellular antioxidants like vitamin C doesn't help. It's like having 10 cash registers in a grocery store with 10 cashiers operating them, increasing the number of cashiers doesn't help the lines move any faster because the rate limiting step is the number of cash registers—NADPH represents the cash registers. The only way to *increase* the ability of antioxidants to neutralize free radicals is to increase the charge of NADPH—and beta-hydroxybutyrate is the only proven way to do that.

Veech and Krebs felt the constant touting of antioxidants by physicians, researchers, health advocates and the food industry was one of the largest sources of misinformation ever propagated to the public. This would also explain why generations of researchers, in an attempt to validate Harmon's Free Radical Theory of Aging, failed to extend the lifespan of animals by feeding them antioxidants.

As Veech stated, perhaps the *only* way to improve the antioxidant function within the cell is through ketosis. In 2017 Veech and his colleagues directly tested the ability of the ketone ester to blunt free radical damage. The study exposed mice to a high dose of ionizing radiation (ionizing radiation splits water, creating free radicals). The results were stunning. Giving the mice a large, single dose of the ketone ester 24 hours after exposure to the radiation "led to a consistent 50 percent decrease in numerous types of radiation-induced chromosomal malformations and abnormal cell divisions." This is also the possible reason why Tour de France riders seem to experience an "unprecedented" ability to recover during the grueling race. The unrelenting physical demand of the Tour demands an extraordinary amount of aerobic energy generation and massive oxygen intake that results in free radical generation. Ingesting the ketone ester could mitigate the overall damage from free radicals resulting in enhanced recovery. "This is perhaps the most unique quality of BHB," said a colleague of Veech.

What about the second source of aging: the slow erosion of our epigenetic software according to Sinclair's theory? Are there ways to slow the pernicious disorganization of the epigenome? Indeed, slowing epigenetic drift would preserve the capacity of stem cells to replace the cells lost to apoptosis. Recent work by Sinclair's group has illuminated why the sirtuin activity essential to maintaining our epigenome declines precipitously with age. Critically, sirtuins require NAD+ as a coenzyme to function. In fact, the level of NAD+ is what's known as the *rate limiting step* in sirtuin activity—its level alone determines how well sirtuins do their job. But here's the rub: levels of NAD+ decline dramatically as we age. Between the ages of 40 and 80 the level of NAD+ declines by about 33 percent. Starved of NAD+, sirtuins lose the ability to repair DNA *and* maintain our epigenome in a youthful state. Fortuitously, researchers have recently discovered ways to help sirtuins do their job more efficiently—to help repair DNA damage *and* maintain the fidelity of the epigenome. Exciting new research on NAD+ precursor supplements (nicotinamide mononucleotide and nicotinamide riboside), largely spearheaded by Sinclair's laboratory, have shown the ability to restore NAD+ back to more youthful levels.

Restoring levels of NAD+, as you can by now imagine, is critical for optimal cellular functionality. In addition to sirtuin function, NAD+ is one of the four "great" controlling coenzymes essential to driving our metabolism.

Veech points out that BHB can maintain youthful levels of NAD+ without NAD+ precursor supplementation. Here's the crux: The main source of NAD+ loss within cells comes from DNA repair enzymes "using up" stores of NAD+. Because ketosis substantially decreases endogenous free radical production, while simultaneously increasing glutathione levels, less NAD+ is consumed by DNA repair enzymes. BHB's ability to raise levels of NAD+ is not just theoretical: feeding rats a ketogenic diet has demonstrated a dramatic increase in NAD+ levels in the brain within just a few days.

Indeed, the life-extending mechanisms triggered by caloric restriction are extravagantly intertwined with the metabolic switch to ketosis. Perhaps Veech was right, the vast spectrum of health promoting effects demonstrated from caloric restriction may be largely due to one molecule: beta-hydroxybutyrate. Given the way evolution operates, this makes sense. In 2003 Veech and Cahill predicted: "A chemical agent, BHB, that has played such a major role in man's survival may be expected to have actions other than simple calories. When nature has a beneficial substance, it may become *pleiotropic* though evolution with survival advantages."

The concept of *pleiotropy* is fascinating. Evolution is a clever engineer. The relentless forward momentum of Darwinian evolution abhors inefficiency. Evolution is forced to paint on a narrow canvas—there is only *so much* storage space in our genome. Over eons, our genomes have unceasingly remodeled themselves, acquiring useful information and discarding outdated information. The disposal of an unnecessary gene frees up storage space within DNA to evolve new genes that may confer a survival advantage, thus increasing odds for reproduction. A compelling example: along the way, we humans lost the gene for vitamin C synthesis. Once we consistently took in enough of it through diet, evolution was free to discard it.

Additionally, in its relentless drive for efficiency, evolution often piggybacks on what is already in place by adding functionality—this is the concept of *pleiotropy*. An example of this is your garage door opener. When you press the button to open your garage door it also triggers a light to come on so you don't stumble through your dark garage. This dual functionality is pleiotropy in action—it is much more efficient to have one button do both jobs than build an entire new system to operate the light. Ongoing research on BHB has proven it to be *extraordinarily* pleiotropic, just as Veech and Cahill predicted in 2003. Recent research has shown that evolution built epigenetic signaling into BHB, providing the signal for longevity genes to turn on.

BHB's epigenetic signaling is due to its ability to inhibit a class of epigenetic proteins called histone deacetylases (HDAC). HDAC proteins turn down the expression of genes by removing certain "ornaments" from histones.

BHB can inhibit HDACs from removing their attachments to histones, thus turning up the dial on the production of associated genes. One of the genes turned up by BHB belongs to a family of proteins called the forkhead box proteins (FOXO). FOXO genes transcribe proteins known as *transcription factors*, epigenetic acting proteins that physically associate themselves with DNA. When FOXO proteins interact with DNA, it alters the expression of hundreds of genes. FOXO proteins instruct DNA to boost internal antioxidant capacity, upregulating production of glutathione and other internal antioxidants like superoxide dismutase and catalase, thus circling back to slowing the ticking clock of the free radical damage that drives aging in the first place. (The addition of superoxide dismutase and catalase increases the cell's antioxidant capacity because they operate through a different mechanism of action than the NADP+ dependent antioxidants.) Furthermore, FOXO is required for stem cell self-renewal, helping to address the second aspect of aging, the slow loss of stem cell function due to epigenetic drift.

Veech's bold assertion that "the lifespan extension produced by caloric restriction can be duplicated by the metabolic changes induced by ketosis" has been addressed in recent studies that have tantalizingly hinted that ketosis may be able to extend lifespan *independent* of caloric restriction as Veech claimed. In 2014, a study demonstrated that the simple addition of BHB to the diet of the nematode, C. *elegans,* increased lifespan by 20 percent. A more comprehensive mouse study followed in 2017. This study compared the effects of a high-carbohydrate control diet, a low-carbohydrate diet, and a ketogenic diet on lifespan. Importantly, the diets were equal in calories so they were compared on the merit of their macronutrient ratios alone. The results suggested a dose dependent effect: median lifespan of mice on the control diet was 886 days compared to 943 for the low-carbohydrate diet, and a stunning 1003 days for the ketogenic diet, an increase of 13 percent. Perhaps Veech had it right: "It's the ketones, stupid."

Today, the remarkable properties of ketone metabolism— once thought to be a dangerous, pathological condition—have captured the attention of researchers around the globe. In 2014, researchers at Yale uncovered another surprising, pleiotropic effect of BHB. They discovered that BHB suppresses activation of the NLRP3 inflammasome (a large, multi-protein complex that initiates inflammation), thus dramatically reducing inflammation. A "surprising" finding by an author of the study that was admittedly "agnostic" about ketone metabolism going into the research.

The Yale researchers then wondered if ketosis might alter other aspects of the immune system. They decided to design a study that asked a specific question: Could ketosis offer protection from a viral infection like influenza? The researchers fed a group of mice a ketogenic diet containing less than 1 percent carbs and a second group a standard mouse chow with 58 percent carbs. They then infected both groups with an influenza virus. The mice in the ketogenic diet group had lower levels of the virus and greater survival rates. The result centered on a specific class of immune cells called gamma delta T cells that were spurred to life in the ketogenic diet group but not in the standard diet group. Gamma delta T cells are responsible for producing mucus in the linings of the lungs, which is a critical first-line defense for the body to rid itself of infectious agents. The job of the mucus is to trap the virus and then travel up the airways where it can be coughed out. "This was a totally unexpected finding," said an author of the study. "We have no idea yet why the gamma delta T cells appear to become activated by the keto diet. This is something we'll be pursuing in the future."

Indeed, some of the evidence in support of ketosis—whether it is induced by fasting, a ketogenic diet, exogenous ketones, MCT oil, or some combination of all four—might be right in front of our eyes. If one takes a quick visual survey across the animal kingdom, virtually every wild species looks healthy—it's impossible to find an obese lion or chimpanzee or deer in their natural habitat. Conversely, as species, we do seem curiously sickly. Obesity, diabetes, depression, cancer and autoimmunity are alarmingly becoming the norm. "Ketosis is a normal physiologic state. I would argue it is the normal state of man. It's not normal to have McDonald's and a delicatessen around every corner. It's normal to starve," said Veech.

If Veech is right, it may offer a singular explanation for our sorry state. Most people in the Western world, it is safe to say, may never experience a prolonged state of ketosis brought on by periods of starvation. Our cheap, carbohydrate dominant diets have effectively smothered this built in therapeutic state that has been with us for millions of years. Today, most Americans will slowly develop insulin resistance and systemic inflammation followed by a progressively less efficient metabolism. Eyesight fades, memories are harder to access, fatigue and apathy set in. Everything is diminished.

The list of pathologies that ketone metabolism has shown promise to treat, and more importantly, *prevent*, is large and growing. From insulin resistance, diabetes, and neurodegeneration, the list has expanded to include cancer and other diseases associated with free-radical production and now, viral infection and critically, *aging*. In time, it is almost inevitable that other diseases with similar etiologies will be added to the list. On some level, it does seem almost too good-to-be-true, and optimistically, it's hard to imagine that the power of ketosis will again be lost to time.

THE FUTURE

How will future generations perceive our current health care system, what we, today, call "modern medicine?" Will they shake their heads in disbelief? Will the flaws seem obvious to them, which today are clouded, murky and unclear to us? Will future generations feel a twinge of empathy for us? Modern medicine, to be sure, has miraculous capabilities that our ancestors would marvel at: Imaging technologies like CT scans and MRIs, robotic-guided surgeries, and artificial intelligence (AI) programs that can diagnose cancer far better than humans can. Yet, even with these advanced technologies that transcend human capabilities, something feels . . . *off*. We can build AI programs that predict the exact molecular architecture needed to design a new drug that docks to a specific receptor, yet 40 percent of the population is obese—and over half are pre-diabetic or diabetic. We can visualize our inner selves with CT scans, ultrasound and MRIs yet depression and anxiety run rampant. Perhaps we've veered off course. Perhaps we have focused on the trees at the expense of the forest—we have favored technology over simplicity and we have lost sight of something critical—the real meaning of health care.

Warburg, Krebs, and Veech, each of a different generation, felt the same thing. All three of them entered the world of clinical medicine as medical doctors and paused. All three felt a visceral pull drawing them to look beyond the known science to something more essential yet elusive. Something fundamental. This shared pull may have been communicated at an unspoken, unconscious level. Yet the desire was translated into something real: the continuum of research—from Warburg to Krebs to Veech—ultimately defined the manifest qualities of ketone metabolism.

Still, the stunning therapeutic potential of ketosis falls into a health care system that has shown little interest in free or dirt-cheap therapies. There is simply no financial incentive for big pharma or physicians to care about low-cost therapies. Unglamorous therapies like fasting, ketogenic diets, or non-patentable ketone supplements attract little money and therefore little attention. The mismatch between the potential value of these therapies and their adoption by the health care system is staggering—it's like valuing Amazon or Apple stock at close to zero. We spend billions annually on chemotherapy drugs that change outcomes by mere weeks or months; billions on stents, statins, bariatric surgeries and diabetes drugs and devices that don't even scratch the surface of the core problems of insulin resistance, diabetes and obesity. Big pharma has spent billions on developing drugs for dementia, Alzheimer's and Parkinson's and have come away empty handed. Yet, we have this incredibly promising, perfectly safe, and incredibly cheap therapy sitting right in front of us that is largely ignored. This frustrated Veech. "He was optimistic that each publication would convince people of the ester's importance, but then he often felt let down," said one of Veech's closest friends. He truly thought the ester could change the world, change the lives of billions of fellow humans for the better. He felt the ester was the "equivalent of the discovery of penicillin. If not bigger." Clarke, the co-developer of the ester, still believes that the ketone ester will eventually be "more or less a general tonic for the general population."

Future generations will most likely be befuddled by our current approach to health care. Strangely, we place each disease into its own little-box and wait until it's entrenched within us, when it's too late, before we attempt to treat it. Physicians surgically rearrange vasculature or insert stents to treat failing arteries. They make futile attempts to salvage a body riddled with cancer by dripping in toxic chemotherapy drugs or burning with radiation. They prescribe insulin shots for people with diabetes, steroids to quell autoimmunity, and so on. But a sober top-down analysis reveals how misguided this purely reactive strategy is. Consider this: if a pill was invented that cured cancer tomorrow, it would only extend the human lifespan by 2.9 years. Why? The unremitting process of entropy will foist some other age-related disease immediately upon us. The same holds true for all other major diseases. According to an analysis performed from scientists at University of Southern California, University of Illinois at Chicago, Harvard, Columbia, and other institutions, "Lowering the incidence of cancer by 25 percent in the next few decades—in line with the most favorable historical trends—would barely improve population health over not doing anything at all. The same is true of heart disease, the leading cause of death worldwide. About the same number of older adults would be alive but disabled in 2060 whether researchers do nothing or continue to combat cancer and heart disease individually." Yet, investing in therapies that combat aging stand to pay *enormous* dividends. According to the analysis, "Even modest success in slowing aging would increase the number of non-disabled older adults by five percent every year from 2030 to 2060." Proof of this is easy to come by: extending the lifespan of mice by caloric restriction postpones *all* age-related diseases. To parse disease up and battle each condition individually is trying to reverse entropy at its zenith—it's a losing game. The efforts of health care should focus on prevention over cure; pharmaceutical research should be redirected toward anti-aging interventions.

Of course the power of prevention is nothing new, but it remains universally true. The well-known adage once quipped by Benjamin Franklin: "An ounce of prevention is worth a pound of cure," is as true today as it was when he first said it in 1736. The idea that a little prevention has much more value than a lot of cure not only makes intuitive sense, it is in harmony with the physical laws of the universe. The second law of thermodynamics states that the universe spontaneously trends toward an increasing amount of disorder, the universal law of entropy. A healthy body has low entropy—it is highly ordered. A body with cardiovascular disease, cancer, or metabolic syndrome, for example, has high entropy, it is rapidly trending toward disorder. Instead of trying to fix the damage while the waters are rising, we should be damming the river. And we know the source of the river. In the world of biology, entropy goes by a different term: *aging*. All of the Western world's leading killers are ultimately caused by the aging process. To address aging is to address virtually every disease process. It's difficult to undo entropy. It is far better to try to preserve order as long as possible. And this, Veech claimed, is precisely what ketone metabolism does—preserve the highly structured order of our bodies, keeping it thrumming along optimally—a sophisticated, internally installed therapy that evolved over eons to keep us healthy and reproducing, fulfilling our Darwinian imperative.

It's worth pointing out that the vast majority of the twentieth and twenty-first century breakthroughs in biology do not come from man inventing something de-novo, they arise from man borrowing nature's intellectual property: genetic engineering, monoclonal antibodies, CRISPR, stem cell induction and cloning; all of these inventions, most of them blessed by a Nobel Prize, are less inventions in the true sense, and more just manipulations of the exquisite biological systems that nature honed over millions of years of evolution. Why reinvent the wheel? And truth be told, we are not yet very good at it. Man-made drugs are typically blunt, clumsy, and indiscriminate. Our attempts to target a specific disease process with drugs almost always come packaged with a litany of unintended side-effects. This is not to say we won't be better at de-novo drug development in the future—we are just not that good at it *yet*. Our attempts to slow entropy in one location speeds it up in others. The totality of healthcare seems more like a game of whack-a-mole against entropy: drugs that attempt to undo arterial plaques and untangle neurofibrillary tangles, surgeries that attempt to "cut out" or "bypass" entropy wherever and whenever it surfaces. Our healthcare system needs to be turned inside-out.

Heeding these lessons from physics, the primary goal of health care should be to preserve our momentary gift of order—prevent entropy as long as possible. To this end, Veech's final message was that we don't need to look too far. We don't need to try to invent something new. We *own* nature's IP. Our bodies have a targeted, preventive-strategy already installed that can be triggered by fasting, a ketogenic diet or by ingesting the ketone ester.

Richard Veech died on February 2, 2020, shortly after addressing an audience of his peers at a conference in New Mexico, or as he might say, his "great" controlling nucleotides reached their final equilibrium. Genius often appears in unusual packages. Those who knew Dr. Veech well universally described him as a colorful character. To be sure, he had little patience for fools. He was refreshingly and, at times, shockingly blunt. He called it exactly how he saw it, using as few words as possible and with little concern for political correctness. "Read the damn papers," he once told a reporter asking him to explain the ketone ester's significance. Although some were obviously put off by his rough edges, others appreciated his straight forward style. Those I interviewed for this book who were close to him, unquestionably loved him. Veech had no interest in fame or self-promotion—in fact, he felt that it was "unseemly for doctors to promote themselves," insisting instead to be judged on the merit of his work alone.

There was another side to Dr. Veech. For those he loved he was gracious and thoughtful, as illustrated in a letter he wrote to the two sons of George Cahill upon Cahill's death: "It is one of my proudest accomplishments to have been cited as a single co-author with Dr. Cahill [on] one of his last publications. Dr. Cahill died at 85 while singing with two of his daughter's Handel's Hallelujah Chorus. I related this to a young student studying ketosis in athletes and she exclaimed 'He must have gone immediately to heaven.' That is an idea that all of us who knew him would share."

The legacy of a scientist is a curious thing. All too often it is not fully appreciated until after they are gone. Many of the scientists in this book: Warburg, Krebs, and Mitchell were fortunate enough to have received recognition in the form of a Nobel Prize while still alive. Although Veech was never awarded a Nobel Prize, in the final analysis time may prove his research—his message—to be just as far reaching. Perhaps even more profound than his predecessors. It is poetic, in a way, that the human side of this story syncs with Veech's professional legacy. Warburg took a chance on Krebs—an inexperienced medical doctor at the time—as did Krebs with Veech. Together, in the end, their combined research wove a tapestry that transcended each of their individual careers and accomplishments. Although awards are given to individual scientists, advancements in science are never an individual achievement. It is a collective effort—a canvas that is filled-in over many generations. Science is the most altruistic and unselfish of human activities—an offering—the gift of free and accumulating knowledge. "If I have seen further it is by standing on the shoulders of giants," said Isaac Newton. And like the transgenerational canvas of science, the first part of Veech's professional legacy revealed our metabolism to be the same: reactions evolving into pathways, evolving over eons into a single, interconnected whole. A lattice of thousands of harmonically connected reactions controlled by the four "great" nucleotide coenzymes. The second pillar of Veech's legacy was revealing the potent therapeutic qualities of the misunderstood and often maligned fuel molecule, beta-hydroxybutyrate. Operating through the four-nucleotide coenzymes, it alone could change the complexion of our entire metabolism in ways that were once thought immutable. The legacy of Veech will continue. The fascinating qualities of BHB are still being uncovered.

Veech's belief in the ketone ester was genuine. In the winter of 2015, with his 55th Harvard reunion fast approaching, Dr. Veech penned a letter to his classmates extolling the virtues of the ketone ester: "As most of us will be entering our 8th decade, far beyond our allotted 3 score and ten, I thought it might be of interest to present to my classmates some of the research findings that have occupied me for the past 20 years concerning the accompaniment of aging." He then listed 10 publications supporting the ester's ability to ameliorate age related cognitive decline.

What does the future hold? What will health care look like in the generations to come? It might feel excruciatingly slow at times, but the vector of human progress is always forward. As physics has taught us, this forward march of societal evolution is baked into the fabric of the universe. It is an extension of the order-seeking eruption of life itself. Gravity is the universal fountain-head of order. The flow of negative entropy from our sun that spurred the formation of life doesn't stop there. Nature repeats patterns. Bear with me for a moment: over three billion years ago life began as a self-replicating molecule. This evolved into a self-replicating cell, which in turn evolved into a self-replicating multicellular organism with individual cells performing tasks for a given system. Multicellular life is a collective, if you will, an economy of divided labor. Evolution is a march up a staircase of functionality, molecules to cells to multicellular organisms. Civilization, too, is repeating this same pattern—marching up this same staircase of functionality. We have gone from caves, to cities, to the industrial revolution, the internet revolution, artificial intelligence and up and up. Science is perhaps the pinnacle of this societal evolution—the universe peering into the innerworkings of itself.

We can *only* get better at medicine in the future—it is *writ large* in the universe. But today the flaws in our health care system are substantial and systemic and will be obvious to future generations. We spend enormous amounts of money overtreating with drugs, procedures and surgeries that don't move the needle on our overall health. Future generations will instead focus on primary, preventative care—health care in harmony with the laws of thermodynamics. Technology will track outcomes. More convenient, at-home blood tests will be developed that encourage engagement, sustainability and a continuum of care. Cell phone apps will store results, allowing for a much more convenient interface between patients and doctors. COVID-19 has hastened the inevitable change to more efficient health care delivery through telemedicine—a system that is more user friendly, leverages technology to remove friction and is better able to facilitate primary, preventive health care. In time, we will get better at warding off the chronic diseases of aging and lengthening our health span. This is not very complicated. It could be implemented now, but we first have to fix the horribly broken incentive structure of our current health care system. If one were able to patent a simple three or four day fast a handful of times per year and put it into pill form, it would almost certainly be a billion-dollar, blockbuster drug. Same with a well-executed ketogenic diet or a quality exogenous ketone supplement administered preventively at midlife or when the first signs insulin resistance surface. The benefits of ketosis are enormous—initiating a cascade of changes that affects our entire metabolism—the chemical motion that quantifies our perception of time and defines our health—the chemical motion that *is* our vital spark. But the good news is that none of us have to wait for the system to catch up. Each of us can be a health care system of one.

https://youtu.be/116WSn2WRLs

IMPLEMENTING KETOSIS INDUCING STRATEGIES

This appendix is by no means intended to be a comprehensive guide to the implementation of a ketogenic diet, fasting protocols, or the best use of MCT oil or exogenous ketone supplementation, but rather a broad survey to point you towards a few of the possible paths to acquire more information. While ketosis can be approached in a variety of ways, or by some combination of the above methods, no one has yet to identify the optimal way to achieve ketosis for a specific goal or condition. To slow aging and prevent disease, is it best to fast intermittently or to eat a strict ketogenic diet? Or is it better in the long run to eat a low-carbohydrate diet and supplement with MCT oil or a ketone ester? Or is it enough to engage in short fasts once or twice a month—or seasonally—and not be concerned about diet? The only way to answer these difficult questions is by rigorous and expensive clinical trials. Nevertheless, even without evidence-based answers to these questions, there are general guidelines that seem to draw on a consensus among the experts.

When should someone consider ketosis inducing strategies (KIS) for antiaging and disease prevention?

Consensus suggests that midlife—or earlier if signs of insulin resistance emerge—is a reasonable time to consider implementing KIS. Of course, this is subjective. An athletic 50-year-old eating a high-carbohydrate diet may have no metabolic dysfunction and remain highly sensitive to insulin. Conversely, someone in their late 20s or early 30s may already be deep in the throes of insulin resistance and metabolic dysfunction.

How do I know if I'm developing insulin resistance or metabolic dysfunction?

Fasting blood glucose readings will often reveal progressive insulin resistance. An even better biomarker is A1C. A1C provides an estimated average blood glucose reading spanning the previous three months. According to the American Diabetes Association an A1C level above 5.7% and less than 6.5% is the prediabetes range and an A1C level of 6.5% or higher is the diabetes range. If you're creeping toward an A1C in the upper 5 percent it may be a good time to implement KIS. Or, if you are entering midlife and wish to proactively push back against the universal law of entropy with the goal of preserving your health as long as possible, you might consider KIS now.

What is the best ketone implementing strategy?
Again, there is no evidence-based, peer-reviewed, consensus answer to this question: it is certain to be highly individualized depending on age, gender, metabolic status, genetics and level of motivation. In terms of difficulty, the ketogenic diet is the most complex with fasting and ketone supplementation the least complex. That is not to say a ketogenic diet can't be incorporated seamlessly into one's life; it just has a steeper learning curve. Successful implementation also depends on one's willingness and ability to make the necessary life adjustments. No expert—to the best of my knowledge— suggests that a ketone supplement or an occasional fast will compensate for a bad diet. However, ketosis-implementing strategies don't have to be so restrictive or difficult that they detract from one's quality of life. For me—a 48-year-old interested in warding off disease and staying healthy as long as possible—I eat in a time-restricted window, take an exogenous ketone supplement and eat a low-carbohydrate diet. On a typical day, I have a cup of black coffee shortly after awakening. Midmorning, I take about 20 ml of a ketone ester followed by my first meal at around 1:00 p.m. and dinner at around 5 or 6 p.m. with a snack or two in-between. A few times a year, I will water-only fast for 3 to 4 days. For me, this routine captures both the overlapping and unique benefits of fasting, a low-carbohydrate diet and ketone supplementation. Depending on my activity level, I may be in ketosis continuously or intermittently. Moreover, taking the ketone ester on an

empty stomach after fasting overnight for around 15 hours boosts my BHB levels into a range typically associated with longer fasts, allowing me to fully benefit from the anti-inflammatory, epigenetic and antioxidant properties of BHB. I don't have to put too much thought into this routine—I get to eat what I enjoy while restricting only the low-quality sugary and starchy foods that make me feel tired and bloated anyway.

Here are a few links to podcasts with Dominic D'Agostino discussing the nuances of ketosis: https://peterattiamd.com/domdagostinoama01/

https://www.youtube.com/watch?v=keSoSyu9m7c

KIS for Alzheimer's and neurodegenerative disease
The studies presented in the previous chapters have demonstrated that KIS holds extraordinary promise as a treatment for Alzheimer's and other neurodegenerative diseases, especially in the early stages, and even more so for prevention. The story of Steve Newport—and the many other Alzheimer's victims that have followed Mary's advice—along with the preclinical and clinical trials performed to date, indicate that ketosis offers tremendous hope for this insidious disease. The Charlie Foundation has a remarkably informative section on their website describing how, when and why to implement KIS for a range of conditions including Alzheimer's, epilepsy, brain tumor/cancer, Parkinson's Disease, traumatic brain injury, mitochondrial disease, autism, ALS and brain health. Visit the site here: https://charliefoundation.org/

Mary Newport's TED talk: https://www.youtube.com/ watch?v=Dvh3JhsrQ0w&index=4&list=PLf3xkKFsZaCgsT 4GB4ruqrl5hmVquxyNB&t=63s

KIS for cancer

For cancer, the ketogenic diet and fasting have demonstrated tremendous promise as adjunctive and neoadjunctive cancer therapies—setting up a beautiful therapeutic differential between the metabolism of cancer cells and healthy cells. To learn more about implementing a ketogenic diet for cancer I highly recommend the book *Keto for Cancer* by Miriam Kalamian EdM MS CNS. The Charlie Foundation website is another great resource. Interest in metabolic therapies for cancer has exploded in recent years and a growing number of researchers are pivoting to this white-hot field of research. Thomas Seyfried at Boston College, Dominic D'Agostino at the University of South Florida and Valter Longo at UCLA are a few of the pioneers in this field and are still actively researching the effects of KIS on cancer. Dr. Longo's research has shown that fasting (or a fasting-mimicking diet) paired with chemotherapy or radiation holds the tremendous potential to mitigate side effects while simultaneously enhancing the efficacy of the therapy. Dr. Seyfried and Dr. D'Agostino's preclinical research has suggested that the ketogenic diet holds the same potential that Longo observed with patients in the clinic. Dr. Seyfried and Dr. D'Agostino are currently researching combinations of metabolic drugs and therapies that synergize with the ketogenic diet. Visit PubMed and search their names to find their latest research. I whole-heartedly believe that synergistic strategies are the way forward for this terrible malady. Nontoxic combinations of metabolic and epigenetic acting therapies offer new hope for cancer patients, and can't come fast enough.

Valter Longo discussing fasting and cancer: https://www.youtube.com/watch?v=LGafhm1cuSI

Thomas Seyfried lecture: https://www.youtube.com/watch?v=KusaU2taxow

KIS for COVID-19

Research has unequivocally established that insulin resistance and diabetes is a potent risk factor for the severity of a COVID-19 infection. Low-carbohydrate diets, ketogenic diets and/or intermittent fasting have proven to be effective ways to reverse the metabolic dysfunction behind insulin resistance. We missed a wonderful opportunity to hammer this message home while most people were quarantined during the initiation stage of the pandemic. Correcting metabolic dysfunction may still be one of the best tools people have to combat COVID-19.

Additionally, there is reason to suspect that ketosis may offer multiple mechanisms of protection from acute respiratory distress syndrome that extend beyond the correction of metabolic dysfunction. Last year's preclinical study conducted at Yale (cited in an earlier chapter) demonstrated that in mice a ketogenic diet can dramatically expand a critically important class of T-cells that trap the influenza virus early in the infection process. Two researchers at the Buck Institute in San Francisco, Brianna Stubbs and John Newman, recently published a review article titled "Investigating Ketone Bodies as Immunometabolic Countermeasures Against Respiratory Viral Infections." The article points out that the drug-like effects of BHB—particularly the ability to reduce inflammation by inhibiting the NLRP3 inflammasome and the neutralization of free radicals by increasing the NADPH to NADP ratio—could reduce the severity of respiratory viral infections. "Basic research shows that BHB directly inhibits the activation of the pro-inflammatory pathway NLRP3, which is central to the disease pathogenesis of COVID-19 and is a likely contributor to the cytokine storm," said Stubbs. Newman and Stubbs—like all great researchers—are extremely cautious in making unsubstantiated claims and are quick to point out that the direct effect of a ketogenic diet or ketone supplementation on COVID-19 is entirely speculative at this point. "I want to be clear that there is no evidence that a ketogenic diet is protective in any way against COVID-19," said Newman. Nevertheless, previously published basic research suggests that BHB supplementation or a ketogenic diet may be a nontoxic and novel treatment strategy to potentially reduce the severity of the illness while also mitigating the worrisome and lingering after effects that are being reported. "Dying is not the only bad outcome from COVID-19. Some survivors are presenting with long-term severe memory impairments, extreme exhaustion and weakness from muscle wasting following an extended time in the hospital," said Newman.

Plans on testing ketosis on COVID-19 are underway. Doctors at Johns Hopkins will place a small group of intubated patients suffering from COVID-19 on a ketogenic diet and measure outcomes. "The hope is that the diet will improve oxygen exchange, reduce the duration of time on ventilators and perhaps most importantly, reduce the systemic inflammation that leads to the cytokine storm that often precedes the development of acute respiratory distress syndrome." In the meantime, there is every reason to be proactive—getting oneself in metabolic shape will not only reap benefits in every aspect of your life—from energy levels, mental clarify to longevity—but it may also be, for now, the best tool we have in our fight against COVID-19.

And, of course, always consult your doctor before taking any supplements or implementing any dietary changes.

REFERENCES

THE VITAL FORCES

Memoirs of the Rev. Dr. Joseph Priestley to the Year 1795, Joseph Priestly, General Books LLC (February 7, 2012)

"Founders Online: From Benjamin Franklin to Joseph Priestley, 19 September 1772." National Archives and Records Administration, National Archives and Records Administration, founders.archives.gov/documents/Franklin/01-19-02-0200.

"Joseph Priestley, Discoverer of Oxygen National Historic Chemical Landmark." American Chemical Society, www.acs.org/content/acs/en/education/whatischemistry/landmarks/josephpriestleyoxygen.html.

Gromov. Introduction Aux mystères. Actes Sud Editions, 2012.

Lavoisier, Antoine Laurent, and Robert Kerr. Elements of Chemistry. By A.L. Lavoisier. (Translated by Robert Kerr.) Analytical Theory of Heat. By Jean Baptiste Joseph Fourier. (Translated by Alexander Freeman.) Experimental Researches in Electricity. By Michael Faraday. Encyclopaedia Britannica, 1952.

Michel de Montaigne, Essais, Simon Millanges, Jean Richer, 1580.

Martha Marquardt, Paul Ehrlich (New York: Schuman, 1951)

Cristi.albu@gmail.com. "PNEUMA AND IGNIS." Greek Medicine: PNEUMA AND IGNIS, www.greekmedicine. net/b_p/Pneuma_and_Ignis.html.

Chintamani Nagesa Ramachandra Rao, Lives and Times of Great Pioneers in Chemistry (lavoisier to Sanger), World Scientific Publishing, 2016

Andrea C Buchholz, Dale A Schoeller, Is a calorie a calorie?, The American Journal of Clinical Nutrition, Volume 79, Issue 5, May 2004, Pages 899S–906S, https://doi. org/10.1093/ajcn/79.5.899S

Hans Krebs, Otto Warburg, Cell Physiologist, Biochemist, Eccentric, Clarendon Press – Oxford, 1981

"Antoine-Laurent Lavoisier." Science History Institute, 11 Dec. 2017, www.sciencehistory.org/historical-profile/antoine-laurent-lavoisier.

The History of Cell Respiration and Cytochrome, David Keilin, Cambridge At The University Press, 1966

Apple, Sam. "An Old Idea, Revived: Starve Cancer to Death." The New York Times, The New York Times, 12 May 2016, www.nytimes.com/2016/05/15/magazine/warburg-effect-an-old-idea-revived-starve-cancer-to-death.html.

"Obituary Notice. David Keilin, 1887–1963." Microbiology, Microbiology Society, 1 Nov. 1966, www.microbiologyresearch.org/content/journal/micro/10.1099/00221287-45-2-159;jsessionid=7U2700Ixdi-IfIvYQ7Y7o_qN.mbslive-10-240-10-57.

Biochemistry: The Chemical Reactions of Living Cells, David Metzler, Academic Press, 1977

LOCATING THE "VITAL SPARK"

Searching for a Mechanism: A History of Cell Bioenergetics, John N. Prebble, Oxford University Press, Jan 3, 2019

Reminiscences and Reflections, Hans Krebs, Oxford University Press; First edition (April 15, 1982)

The oxygen-transferring ferment of respiration, Otto Warburg, Nobel Lecture, December 10, 1931
Hans Krebs: Volume 1: The Formation of a Scientific Life, 1900-1933, Frederic Laurence Holmes, Oxford University Press; 1 edition (December 5, 1991)

Franz Knoop, Oxydationen im Tierkdrper (Stuttgart: Ferdinand Enke, 1931)

Luca, Jacob Whaler (October 12, 2015)

"Obituary Notice. David Keilin, 1887–1963." Microbiology, Microbiology Society, 1 Nov. 1966, www.microbiologyresearch.org/content/journal/micro/10.1099/00221287-45-2-159;jsessionid=7U2700Ixdi-IfIvYQ7Y7o_qN.mbslive-10-240-10-57.

ANTIESTABLISHMENT CHEMISTRY

Wandering in the Gardens of the Mind: Peter Mitchell and the Making of Glynn, John Prebble and Bruce Weber, Oxford University Press; 1 edition (February 27, 2003)

Power, Sex, Suicide: Mitochondria and the meaning of life, Nick Lane, Oxford; 2 edition (October 24, 2018)

Letter, Efraim Racker to E. C. Slater, 7 August 1973.

Nobel Lecture, 1997, John Walker, ATP Synthesis by Rotary Catalysis.

Interview, Young Ko

Edward C. Slater, "Peter Dennis Mitchell, 29 September 1920-10 April 1992," Biographical Memoirs of Fellozos of the Royal Society 40 (1994)

David Keilin's Respiratory Chain Concept and its Chemiosmotic Consequences. Peter Mitchell, Nobel Lecture, 8 December, 1978

The Gene: An Intimate History, Siddhartha Mukherjee, Scribner; Reprint edition (May 2, 2017)

THE "GREAT" CONTROLLING NUCLEOTIDE COENZYMES

Veech, Richard L. "The Determination of the Redox States and Phosphorylation Potential in Living Tissues and Their Relationship to Metabolic Control of Disease Phenotypes." IUBMB, John Wiley & Sons, Ltd, 3 Nov. 2006, iubmb.onlinelibrary.wiley.com/doi/full/10.1002/bmb.2006.49403403168.

Veech RL;Todd King M;Pawlosky R;Kashiwaya Y;Bradshaw PC;Curtis W; "The 'Great' Controlling Nucleotide

Coenzymes." IUBMB Life, U.S. National Library of Medicine, pubmed.ncbi.nlm.nih.gov/30624851/.

Veech, interview Dave Asprey Podcast

Interview, College roommate

Interview, Bill Curtis

THE HERO

"Hanover, NH Moose Mountain Plane Crash, Oct 1968." Hanover, NH Moose Mountain Plane Crash, Oct 1968 | GenDisasters ... Genealogy in Tragedy, Disasters, Fires, Floods Page 1, www.gendisasters.com/new-hampshire/2397/hanover-nh-moose-mountain-plane-crash-oct-1968?page=0%2C3.

"Richard L. Veech Plane Crash Hero (The Decatur Herald, 29 October 1968, Tues; Page 3) [1 of 2]." Newspapers.com, www.newspapers.com/clip/22737250/richard-l-veech-plane-crash-hero-the/.

THE FOURTH FUEL

Of Medicine: In Eight Books, Aulus Cornelius Celsus

Autobiography of Mark Twain, Mark Twain, University of California Press, 1997

Shorvon, S. D., et al. The Treatment of Epilepsy. John Wiley & Sons Inc., 2016.

Wheless, James W. "History of the Ketogenic Diet." Wiley Online Library, John Wiley & Sons, Ltd, 4 Nov. 2008, onlinelibrary.wiley.com/doi/full/10.1111/j.1528-1167.2008.01821.x.

Mudd, Efrain. "The Ketogenic Diet - Ketogenic Diet." Pharmacological Sciences, 24 Aug. 2019, www.pharmaco-logicalsciences.us/ketogenic-diet/the-ketogenic-diet.html.

"Formation of Ketone Bodies." British Medical Journal, U.S. National Library of Medicine, 28 Mar. 1942, www.ncbi.nlm.nih.gov/pmc/articles/PMC2159952/?page=1.

Principles of Biochemistry (second edition), Lehninger, Nelson, Cox, Worth Publisher, 1993

Owen, Oliver E. "Ketone Bodies as a Fuel for the Brain during Starvation." IUBMB, John Wiley & Sons, Ltd, 3 Nov. 2006, iubmb.onlinelibrary.wiley.com/doi/full/10.1002/bmb.2005.49403304246.

Cahill, George F, and Richard L Veech. "Ketoacids? Good Medicine?" Transactions of the American Clinical and Climatological Association, American Clinical and Climatological Association, 2003, www.ncbi.nlm.nih.gov/pmc/articles/PMC2194504/.

Cahill, George F. "Fuel Metabolism in Starvation." Annual Reviews, www.annualreviews.org/doi/10.1146/annurev. nutr.26.061505.111258.

Sato K;Kashiwaya Y;Keon CA;Tsuchiya N;King MT;Radda GK;Chance B;Clarke K;Veech RL; "Insulin, Ketone Bodies, and Mitochondrial Energy Transduction." FASEB Journal : Official Publication of the Federation of American Societies for Experimental Biology, U.S. National Library of Medicine, pubmed.ncbi.nlm.nih.gov/7768357/.

Veech RL;Todd King M;Pawlosky R;Kashiwaya Y;Bradshaw PC;Curtis W; "The 'Great' Controlling Nucleotide Coenzymes." IUBMB Life, U.S. National Library of Medicine, pubmed.ncbi.nlm.nih.gov/30624851/.

Veech, Richard L., et al. "Ketone Bodies, Potential Therapeutic Uses." IUBMB, John Wiley & Sons, Ltd, 3 Jan. 2008, iubmb.onlinelibrary.wiley.com/doi/abs/10.1080/152165401753311780.

Veech RL. The therapeutic implications of ketone bodies: the effects of ketone bodies in pathological conditions: ketosis, ketogenic diet, redox states, insulin resistance, and mitochondrial metabolism. Prostaglandins Leukot Essent Fatty Acids. 2004;70(3):309 319. doi:10.1016/j.plefa.2003.09.007

Veech, Richard L. "The Determination of the Redox States and Phosphorylation Potential in Living Tissues and Their Relationship to Metabolic Control of Disease Phenotypes." IUBMB, John Wiley & Sons, Ltd, 3 Nov. 2006, iubmb.onlinelibrary.wiley.com/doi/pdf/10.1002/bmb.2006.49403403168.

Taubes, Gary. "What If It's All Been a Big Fat Lie?" The New York Times, The New York Times, 7 July 2002, www.nytimes.com/2002/07/07/magazine/what-if-it-s-all-been-a-big-fat-lie.html.

"Military Development of Ketone Esters for Enhancing Performance Ft. Joe Bielitzki: H.V.M.N. Podcast." H.V.M.N., hvmn.com/blogs/podcast/episode-67-military-development-of-ketone-esters-for-enhancing-performance-ft-joe-bielitzki.

Nih. "Development of Ketone Ester Diets." Grantome, NIH, grantome.com/grant/NIH/Z01-AA000112-01.

IT WAS LIKE A LIGHTBULB TURNED ON

Newport, Mary. "My Husband, Alzheimer's Patient." The Atlantic, Atlantic Media Company, 10 Feb. 2012, www.theatlantic.com/health/archive/2012/02/my-husband-alzheimers-patient/252595/.

Mary Newport, Interview with the author.

"073: Dr. Mary Newport - Using Ketones to Combat Brain Inflammation Plus New Recommendations for Alzheimer's." Dr. Anthony Gustin, 23 Aug. 2019, dranthonygustin.com/073-ketones-brain-inflammation/.

Groot, Stefanie de, et al. "Fasting Mimicking Diet as an Adjunct to Neoadjuvant Chemotherapy for Breast Cancer in the Multicentre Randomized Phase 2 DIRECT Trial." Nature News, Nature Publishing Group, 23 June 2020, www.nature.com/articles/s41467-020-16138-3.

Raffaghello L;Safdie F;Bianchi G;Dorff T;Fontana L;Longo VD; "Fasting and Differential Chemotherapy Protection in Patients." Cell Cycle (Georgetown, Tex.), U.S. National Library of Medicine, pubmed.ncbi.nlm.nih.gov/21088487/.

Groot, Stefanie de, et al. "Fasting Mimicking Diet as an Adjunct to Neoadjuvant Chemotherapy for Breast Cancer in the Multicentre Randomized Phase 2 DIRECT Trial." Nature News, Nature Publishing Group, 23 June 2020, www.nature.com/articles/s41467-020-16138-3.

https://www.virtahealth.com/outcomes

Cary, Tom. "Tour De France Riders Ready to Fuel up on Ketones – the Mysterious Energy Drink Developed at Oxford University." The Telegraph, Telegraph Media Group, 5 July 2018, www.telegraph.co.uk/

cycling/2018/07/05/tour-de-france-riders-ready-fuel-ketones-mysterious-energy/.

"What Are Ketones and Why Are the Tour De France's Top Teams Using Them?" Canadian Cycling Magazine, 17 July 2019, cyclingmagazine.ca/sections/news/what-are-ketones-and-why-are-the-tour-de-frances-top-teams-using-them/.

Witts, James. "Understanding Ketones: What Does the Wonder Drink Actually Do?" Cyclingnews.com, Cyclingnews, 12 Feb. 2020, www.cyclingnews.com/features/understanding-ketones-what-does-the-wonder-drink-actually-do/.

Jonny Long. "Questions Raised over Use of Ketone 'Miracle Drink' at Tour De France." Cycling Weekly, 16 July 2019, www.cyclingweekly.com/news/racing/tour-de-france/questions-raised-use-ketone-miracle-drink-tour-de-france-431463#:~:text=Tour%20de%20France-,Questions%20raised%20over%20use%20of%20ketone,drink'%20at%20Tour%20de%20France&text=Jumbo%2DVisma's%20team%20boss%20Richard,so%20far%20won%20four%20stages.

Poffé, Chiel, et al. "Ketone Ester Supplementation Blunts Overreaching Symptoms during Endurance Training Overload." The Journal of Physiology, John Wiley and

Sons Inc., June 2019, www.ncbi.nlm.nih.gov/pmc/articles/ PMC6851819/.

Evans, Mark, et al. "Intermittent Running and Cognitive Performance after Ketone Ester Ingestion." Medicine and Science in Sports and Exercise, U.S. National Library of Medicine, pubmed.ncbi.nlm.nih.gov/29944604/.

"How Ketones Can Combat Alzheimer's." Alzheimers.net, 23 July 2019, www.alzheimers.net/ how-ketones-can-combat-alzheimers/.

Phillips, Matthew C L, et al. "Low-Fat versus Ketogenic Diet in Parkinson's Disease: A Pilot Randomized Controlled Trial." Movement Disorders : Official Journal of the Movement Disorder Society, John Wiley and Sons Inc., Aug. 2018, www.ncbi.nlm.nih.gov/pmc/articles/PMC6175383/.

Cunnane, Stephen C, et al. "Can Ketones Help Rescue Brain Fuel Supply in Later Life? Implications for Cognitive Health during Aging and the Treatment of Alzheimer's Disease." Frontiers in Molecular Neuroscience, Frontiers Media S.A., 8 July 2016, www.ncbi.nlm.nih.gov/pmc/ articles/PMC4937039/.

Mujica-Parodi, Lilianne R., et al. "Diet Modulates Brain Network Stability, a Biomarker for Brain Aging, in Young Adults." PNAS, National Academy of Sciences, 17 Mar. 2020, www.pnas.org/content/117/11/6170.

Peters, R. "Ageing and the Brain." Postgraduate Medical Journal, BMJ Group, Feb. 2006, www.ncbi.nlm.nih.gov/pmc/articles/PMC2596698/.

"It's the Ketones Stupid"

Power, Sex, Suicide: Mitochondria and the meaning of life, Nick Lane, Oxford; 2 edition (October 24, 2018)

Shimazu T;Hirschey MD;Newman J;He W;Shirakawa K;Le Moan N;Grueter CA;Lim H;Saunders LR;Stevens RD;Newgard CB;Farese RV;de Cabo R;Ulrich S;Akassoglou K;Verdin E; "Suppression of Oxidative Stress by β-Hydroxybutyrate, an Endogenous Histone Deacetylase Inhibitor." Science (New York, N.Y.), U.S. National Library of Medicine, pubmed.ncbi.nlm.nih.gov/23223453/.

Roberts, Megan N, et al. "A Ketogenic Diet Extends Longevity and Healthspan in Adult Mice." Cell Metabolism, U.S. National Library of Medicine, 5 Sept. 2017, www.ncbi.nlm.nih.gov/pmc/articles/PMC5609489/.

Veech RL;Bradshaw PC;Clarke K;Curtis W;Pawlosky R;King MT; "Ketone Bodies Mimic the Life Span Extending Properties of Caloric Restriction." IUBMB Life, U.S. National Library of Medicine, pubmed.ncbi.nlm.nih.gov/28371201/.

Gopinath, Suchitra D, et al. "FOXO3 Promotes Quiescence in Adult Muscle Stem Cells during the Process of Self-Renewal." Stem Cell Reports, Elsevier, 20 Mar. 2014, www.ncbi.nlm.nih.gov/pmc/articles/PMC3986584/.

Lifespan: Why We Age—and Why We Don't Have To, David Sinclair, Atria Books; 1 edition (September 10, 2019)

MHS conference, 2018, Keynote.

Youm, Yun-Hee, et al. "The Ketone Metabolite β-Hydroxybutyrate Blocks NLRP3 Inflammasome–Mediated Inflammatory Disease." Nature News, Nature Publishing Group, 16 Feb. 2015, www.nature.com/articles/nm.3804.

Goldberg, Emily L., et al. "Ketogenic Diet Activates Protective Γδ T Cell Responses against Influenza Virus Infection." Science Immunology, Science Immunology, 15 Nov. 2019, immunology.sciencemag.org/content/4/41/eaav2026.

Rauf, ByDon, et al. "Can the Keto Diet Help Fight the Flu?: Everyday Health." EverydayHealth.com, www.everyday-health.com/cold-flu/can-the-keto-diet-help-fight-the-flu/.

THE FUTURE

Interview, College Roommate

Apple, Story by Sam. "The Keto Diet's Most Controversial Champion." The Atlantic, Atlantic Media Company, 6 Nov. 2019, www.theatlantic.com/health/archive/2019/11/patrick-arnold-ketones-baseball-balco/601399/.

Rosales, Lani. "Incredible Fuel Could Treat Countless Diseases, If Only It Was Funded." The American Genius, 28 Aug. 2016, theamericangenius.com/business-news/ketone-ester-fuel-treats-diseases/.

Wu, Suzanne. "Delayed Aging Is Better Investment than Cancer, Heart Disease Research." USC News, 5 June 2014, news.usc.edu/55969/delayed-aging-is-better-investment-than-cancer-heart-disease-research/.

IMPLIMENTING KETOSIS INDUCING STRAGITIES

"Researchers Outline Strategy for Testing Ketone Bodies against COVID-19." ScienceDaily, ScienceDaily, 15 July 2020, www.sciencedaily.com/releases/2020/07/200715131230.htm.

Printed in Great Britain
by Amazon